MANHATTAN PUBLIC LIBRARY DISTRICT

W9-AMB-281

NO GYM REQUIRED ™

IFEB 11 2009

NO GYM REQUIRED™

UNLEASH YOUR INNER ROCKSTAR

JENNIFER COHEN

WITH SUZANNE BOYD

KEY PORTER BOOKS

MANHATTAN PUBLIC LIBRARY DIST.

FEB 11 2009

Copyright © 2009 by Jennifer Cohen

All rights reserved. No part of this work covered by the copyrights hereon may be reproduced or used in any form or by any means—graphic, electronic or mechanical, including photocopying, recording, taping or information storage and retrieval systems—without the prior written permission of the publisher, or, in case of photocopying or other reprographic copying, a licence from Access Copyright, the Canadian Copyright Licensing Agency, One Yonge Street, Suite 1900, Toronto, Ontario, M6B 3A9.

Library and Archives Canada Cataloguing in Publication

Cohen, Jennifer

    No gym required : unleash your inner rockstar / Jennifer Cohen ; with Suzanne Boyd.

ISBN 978-1-55470-110-0

    1. Physical fitness. 2. Nutrition. 3. Health. 4. Motivation (Psychology).
I. Boyd, Suzanne, 1963- II. Title.

RA784.C635 2009   613   C2008-902368-4

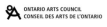

The publisher gratefully acknowledges the support of the Canada Council for the Arts and the Ontario Arts Council for its publishing program. We acknowledge the support of the Government of Ontario through the Ontario Media Development Corporation's Ontario Book Initiative.

We acknowledge the financial support of the Government of Canada through the Book Publishing Industry Development Program (BPIDP) for our publishing activities.

Key Porter Books Limited
Six Adelaide Street East, Tenth Floor
Toronto, Ontario
Canada M5C 1H6
www.keyporter.com

Interior photography: David Wile
Hair and makeup: John Sheehy/Sherrida

Design: Martin Gould
Electronic Formatting: Alison Carr

Printed and bound in Canada
08 09 10 11 12 6 5 4 3 2 1

3 8001 00085 1299

For the Inner rock star in all of us and…

To my late father Michael—you're missed everyday. Thank you so very much for giving me the opportunity to self-actualize. I truly wouldn't have been able to do any of it without your selfless nature and immense generous heart. I love you!

And to my over protective mom. Even though I might not always show it, I appreciate all of it. I love you very much!

CONTENTS

SETTING THE STAGE FOR THE BIG SHOW 9

WHAT YOU WAITING FOR? 19

THE GREATEST LOVE OF ALL 33

ROCK YOUR BODY 71

PART 1: ULTIMATE CARDIO 75

PART 2: POWER MOVES 85

PART 3: 14-DAY ROCK STAR BOOT CAMP 134

ROCK STAR 141

THE NO GYM REQUIRED MENU PLAN 151

ACKNOWLEDGMENTS 187

WORK SHEETS 188

CHAPTER 1

SETTING THE STAGE FOR THE BIG SHOW

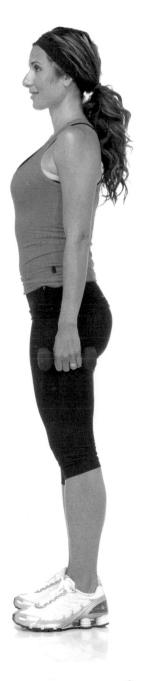

YOU. YES, I AM WRITING THIS BOOK FOR *YOU*, the woman who looks at herself in the mirror and is not satisfied with her body. Instead, she compares herself negatively to the Elle MacPhersons of the world. The Giselle types, who are long and lean, say, 10 feet 6 inches tall, with bodies so seemingly perfect that they appear to be genetic mutations of the most beautiful kind. I am writing this for you, the woman who looks at the covers of those celebrity weeklies while in the supermarket checkout line and wonders why she isn't as thin as this or that "it" girl. You know, those feeble-figured celebs du jour who look 2 pounds soaking wet, each more emaciated than the last. Their "it" look is most likely due to substance abuse with a side order of starvation. And I am writing this book for you, the woman who has marveled at the miraculous transformations of celebrities who go from flab to fab, the ones who lose 30 pounds in 10 days and claim to have done it through a balanced diet and exercise, and is crushed that she is unable to achieve similar results.

I am also writing this book because I am sick and tired of women feeling down about their natural shape, their God-given body type. I am sick and tired of women feeling inadequate, never quite good enough, and striving to look like the images of the models and actresses they see in magazines. More often than not, these celebrities have dieted and exercised—with possible surgical intervention—within an inch of their lives specifically for the photo shoot you so admire, the film they are promoting, or that triumphant walk down the red carpet. Then, of course, there is the artful posing and flattering lighting followed by re-touching, airbrushing, and photo-shopping. In reality, these women themselves often do not measure up to the standards of perfection they represent—standards impossible to maintain in any real-life, real-world scenario.

Now don't get me wrong. I'm not saying be happy with yourself no matter how out of shape you are. Quite the contrary, as being out of shape is unhealthy for the mind, the body, and the soul. Instead, you should want to be in the best possible shape for *you*, which begs the question: Just how perfect are we expected to be? Britney Spears was excoriated for getting jiggly with it in her infamous MTV "comeback," but it is important to note that even when off her honed-to-perfection teen-queen game, she looks better in a bikini than most, even those who are not recent mothers of two. Or, as Jennifer Love Hewitt so brilliantly blogged after being ridiculed for weight gain and cellulite after photos surfaced of her in a bikini: "A size 2 is not fat! Nor will it ever be. And being a size 0 does not make you beautiful. I love my body. To all girls with butts, boobs, hips and a waist, put on a bikini—put it on and stay strong!"

Amen to that, and to the fact that several other young female celebrities came out in Jennifer's support and against this new enter-tainment category that seems to specialize in criticizing so-called figure flaws. Ironically, Hewitt landed the cover of *People Magazine*, quite the *coup* for her troubles, but the magazine industry has been complicit in setting these impossible standards. For example, the Web site Jezebel.com (subtitled "Celebrity, Sex, Fashion without Retouching") caused a brouhaha when it exposed the "before retouching" and "after retouch-ing" images of a Faith Hill *Redbook* cover. The size of the naturally slim singer's waist and arms had been reduced, although they were by no means big to begin with, as was some flesh that peeked over the top of her dress. And even *Glamour*, a magazine well known for championing "real" women, featured a cover shot of a suspiciously streamlined Amer-ica Ferrera, which is ironic considering the actress first achieved renown for embracing her curves and later super-stardom as the "love yourself as you are" icon, "Ugly Betty."

Although this barrage of undermining images originated in the entertainment and fashion worlds of Hollywood and New York, they know no borders and have become relentless, reaching critical mass. It's been estimated that young women are now exposed to 700 fashion and entertainment images a day. *A day!* For this we can thank the Internet explosion, which has sped up our consumption of information. It's more, more, more to feed the 24-hour celebrity news spin cycle. It's a double whammy with magazines having their own Web sites, and a triple threat as the TMZ.coms and PerezHilton.coms of the world have made celebrity a global spectator sport that feeds our unhealthy obsession with their looks and weight.

It goes further and has actually infiltrated our real lives. Take, for instance, the Size Zero syndrome. When actresses started becoming smaller and smaller, we women wanted to do the same. Then the fashion industry jumped onboard to fan the flames. It introduced this so-called size because it fed into the aspirations and was therefore good marketing. But let's think about it for a second. It is impossible to be a size 0 because that would be no size at all! The losers here are women who must now contend with the fact that, as Jennifer Love Hewitt pointed out, a size 2 is considered fat. It's just crazy. I remember when a size 4 was considered tiny. And it is.

The conditioning we women have undergone by the fashion/ entertainment/media complex has led us to desperately want to be everything that most of us are not. But without the Dolly Parton makeover (high hair, high heels, and a plastic surgeon on speed dial) a woman of average height, say, 5 foot 5 inches and with a normally proportioned body at a medically sound weight, will never look like a 5-foot-11-inch supermodel with breasts the size of China and the hips and thighs of a teenage boy! Those genetic rarities are just that—rarities—which is why they are paid obscene amounts of money to stand around and look pretty and—oh yes—thin. Even normal-looking celebrities are put through the thin cycle with all the tricks of the image-making trade.

Some celebrities who realize that their idealized images perpetuate a vicious cycle for women who, in response, try to achieve the unachievable, have told the truth. Tyra Banks eschewed high-fashion modeling for a more lucrative and fame-making commercial career because she decided it was unhealthy to maintain the restrictive weight requirements. Now she uses her hit daytime talk show as a "get real" platform and has televised her unretouched lingerie shots, gleefully pointing out her cellulite and belly fat. When the tabloids targeted her for her 30-pound weight gain, she fought back by appearing on her show in the same swimsuit she was photographed in to prove that she was, in fact, a normal size for a woman of her height.

Kate Winslet has complained publicly when magazines have used technology to drastically slim and lengthen her body. Jennifer Garner never let herself get too thin despite the arduous 4 a.m. workouts and restrictive eating for the action roles that made her famous, and has admitted the level of fitness she achieved for these roles is impossible to maintain over time. But despite the few glimpses behind the curtain—such as those "gotcha" shots of celebrity cellulite that sometimes appear in the tabloids—women en masse buy into the optical illusion of celebrity perfection and, conversely their own "imperfections."

We owe an early debt to Jamie Lee Curtis, an early "activist" who was famed for the *uber*-aerobicized body she achieved for the film *Perfect*, which documented the early 1980s "go-for-the-burn" trend. Fed up with the dream-weaving and the unrealistic expectations of women, she posed for *More Magazine* in her underwear with her "real" tummy. Yes, there were spare tires, and her "real" thighs were exposed in all their unretouched glory. Naturally there was a media storm over her "shocking" and "brave" revelations. Now she is defiantly gray, refusing to color her hair to mask the aging process.

Common sense and human physiology alone tell us that an over-40 celeb with the muscle tone of a 25-year-old has had a little more help than dumbbells and protein shakes, but still we bemoan that our thighs aren't as toned as hers. And when celebrities gain weight, they seem able to bounce back into shape, just like that. And even though we know that it takes a village—Sarah Jessica Parker has admitted that it would have been impossible to regain her "Sex and the City" svelte, post-baby body without her trainer, yoga instructor, nutritionist, and nanny—we judge ourselves for our inability to do the same.

Even I, a fitness person with a degree in psychology, have not been immune to this syndrome. I grew up in Winnipeg, loving food and loving to eat, in a family that socialized around it. And I still do. I have the type of body that I think most women would relate to, one that is fairly normal and real, and that can look average or exceptional depending on the lifestyle choices I make. As a teenager I knew I had to be active to offset the pleasure I derived from food.

I moved to L.A. a decade ago and held several corporate positions in the entertainment industry before realizing that health, wellness, and helping others achieve their personal best was my passion. I moved into fitness.

Despite living in the belly of the beast, L.A. was one of the best things that could have happened to my self-esteem. Not only did I have a bird's-eye view of the unhealthy and self-destructive extremes that the starlets and bona-fide stars would go to in order to achieve the faux fitness that sells, but being surrounded by the skinny-minnies and the skinny-amazons led me to a revelation. Not only was I different in the way I look, I was singular in my commitment to true health through proper and proven practices. I was also different in my approach and philosophy which was and still is, achieving real mental peace through the balance of self-acceptance. Everything going on around me—the starving, the surgery, the all-round self abuse—was against my principles, so it was therefore impossible to compare myself to it. So I just did me. And it worked.

I keep true to realistic goal setting, sustainable results, vigorous training style, and clean eating rules. My degree in psychology allows me to understand the mental needs of my clients and how best to get and keep them motivated. My reputation as a fitness and health expert stayed true to my principles, as I trained and provided nutritional and motivational coaching to record companies, studio execs, and celebrities. Now, after reams of press and media appearances, hundreds of clients, and as a spokesperson for numerous national campaigns for clothing lines and food companies, it's time for me to focus on others.

With *No Gym Required: Unleash your inner Rock Star*, I intend to stop the nonviable and harmful preoccupation women have with wanting to be something they are not and the unhealthy practices they succumb to in attempting to do so. This book will give you the tools to define and then reach the right goals for you. Let's make our plan to turn the celebrity paradigm on its head and make it work for *you*.

Just think, the positive side of being a celebrity must be a wonderfully empowering experience as you are loved and admired, with your needs catered to in the most expert of ways. Imagine how you would feel if you had that type of positive reinforcement in your life every day. And you can, by giving it to yourself. Become your own celebrity, the star of your own world. And not just any type of celebrity. I have always admired rock stars—the way they ooze confidence, their I'm "it" bravado, whatever they happen to look like and however they broadcast the essence of who they are. So here is my first tip for achieving optimum fitness and health—think of yourself as the Rock Star of your own life.

Now this may seem a bit counterintuitive. Traditionally, rock stars have been associated with debauchery and excess—the whole sex, drugs, and rock 'n' roll thing—but being early adopters, rock stars often are first to jump on lifestyle trends that later sweep society. Think of The Beatles and meditation in the 1960s, and Madonna and yoga in the 1990s. Today's most successful and enduring rock stars work out, watch what they eat, and get all the rest they need because they know this is the only route to maintain their best self. The indefatigable Mick Jagger is a well-known "my-body-is-a-temple" type, as is Sheryl Crow. It is perhaps Jennifer Lopez who best exemplifies what I am talking about—the Rock Star mindset that I refer to as "Believe it, achieve it."

Let's look at what she started with—physical attributes that in Hollywood and fashion are not just considered so-so, but major negatives: Smaller breasts, an unusually long waist, and a famously large and wide rear-end. In fact, she is an extreme example of the "dreaded" pear shape that fashion magazines keep showing women how to minimize. But what did JLo do? She hit the gym and the dance studio and literally worked her saddle bags off—she had those as well—turning her body into the best possible version of itself. Then she flaunted her well-toned, but still outsized asset (pun intended) in a series of eye-popping ensembles that not only made her a fashion icon, but made well-padded posteriors chic. And, she did not get breast implants. Then she became a Rock Star.

It can be done and you will do it too. Remember that from now on, you have attained Rock Star status in your own right. I am with your band. Consider this book our tour.

No Gym Required is about a total mindset shift from negative, or just plain neutral, to positive: It is about a focused lifestyle change, but before you can make the transition, you must acknowledge that there are certain baseline requirements for a hit. Think of these as your "general concert rider." Just as JLo has to have white candles and flowers in her dressing room, there's no negotiating on these:

1. Admit that success isn't made overnight. Instead, prepare to work hard, yet more effectively.

2. Eliminate inconsistency. Commit to being consistent with your diet and workout habits.

3. Ditch the unhealthy eating habits —this is 70 percent of the battle.

4. Erase negative mental body images of yourself. Think of yourself as a fit individual.

5. Abolish poor sleeping habits. Regular sleep is key for being able to attack every day with energy.

6. Stop beating yourself up about past mistakes. Yesterday has passed. It's what you do today that sets you up for success tomorrow.

7. Believe you can do it. Believe in your inner Rock Star.

8. Now that you are on the line to the very best possible version of yourself, No Gym Required will take you through:

   - *Goal Setting:* Setting realistic goals to achieve chart-topping success along with how to deal with setbacks and celebrate results.

   - *Smart Eating 101:* You'll learn everything you need including: the star foods and grocery shopping tactics; tips for deciphering food labels; how to distill the protein-fat-carbohydrate debate; what the natural energy and beauty boosters are; how to use herbs and spices as secret weight-loss weapons; the importance of water; ways to maximize weight loss by eating to lose weight and celebrating with a weekly cheat day, plus healthy, tasty, and easy to prepare recipes made with easy-to-find ingredients.

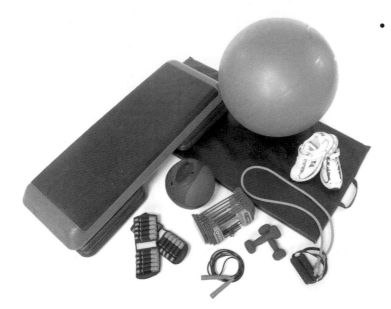

- *Power Moves:* You'll learn my "no gym required" method, which includes a basic tool kit apparatus to allow you to work out anywhere, and uses the most effective multi-functional exercises that maximize results in the minimum amount of time. These will let you "rock your body" whether you are exercising at home or on the road. There are lots of photos in this section to help guide you through to Gold, Platinum, and Double-Platinum status.

Rock Star Fitness gets you an exclusive backstage pass to:

Realistic goals
Optimum information
Confidence to commit to yourself
Kick-ass, back-to-basics training

Strategic lifestyle choices
Tools to think it, live it, be it
Aspiration to be the best possible you
Real-life solutions

Fun
Inspiration
Top-notch psychological insight
Nutrition for health, weight loss, and pleasure
Expert opinion and analysis
Sensible advice
Sustainable results

- *A 14-Day Program:* In this chapter you'll get an easy-to-understand, concise outline of how to start and continue in 14-day segments, implementing the smart eating and power moves information you've learnt in previous chapters. You'll learn about the right mix of cardio and resistance training, how to make interval training work to your advantage, as well as the all-important rest day.

- *A Day in the Life of You, the Rock Star:* Here, you'll be given all my personal tips & tricks, and lists to get you through a typical day, rocking it out with the best snacks and tricks to circumvent overeating pitfalls, travel necessities, shoe-selection guidelines, ways to relax and release stress, and my favorite play lists with songs that keep me revved up while working out. Always remember I'm not only your No Gym Required tour manager, I'm also your biggest fan.

TEAM JENNIFER

No rock star is complete without her entourage or, as the industry likes to call it, team. For some, the team consists of the roadies, manager, agent, lawyer, and accountant. For you, your team begins with your fitness trainer and motivational coach, me! Now allow me to introduce you to two experts, a psychologist and a nutritionist, who will make up the rest of your team. They are essential to this process and like me, will be with you every step of the way as you transform into the best possible you.

First, meet Dr. Leslie Reisner, a clinical psychologist in private practice in Los Angeles, who is also considered one of North America's leading experts in Rational Emotive Behavior Therapy. This form of cognitive-behavioral psychotherapy focuses on identifying and changing behavior that can sabotage a fuller experience of life. In the following chapters, Dr. Reisner will give you effective strategies to stop focusing on the negative, mental exercises to help you get and stay motivated, effective ways to avoid the inevitable temptations and pitfalls, and how best to deal with them if and when you succumb. Dr. Reisner received her bachelor of science degree in psychology from Cornell University, her master of science degree in experimental psychology from Villanova University, and both her master of arts degree and doctorate degree in clinical psychology from Hofstra University. She received her clinical training at the world-famous Institute for Rational Emotive Behavior Therapy (REBT) in New York City under Albert Ellis, Ph.D., the founder of REBT and the 1996 recipient of an award acknowledging his significant contribution to the field of psychology. Along with regular appearances in the print and electronic media, Dr. Reisner lectures and leads numerous workshops on stress management, overcoming eating and other addictive disorders, and fostering emotional intelligence, amongst other topics. Dr. Reisner also teaches continuing education courses in stress management at UCLA and Phillip's Graduate Institute.

Also on your team is Amy Snider PHEc. Amy is a professional food expert who specializes in developing nutritious recipes. Amy's were the perfect choice to assist me in creating delicious recipes to compliment the 14-day menu plan. As Vice President of Sensory Excellence with Dana McCauley & Associates Ltd., a leading consulting company to the food industry, Amy has developed nutrition programs and guided food marketers to use health and diet messages responsibly and meaningfully. Amy has been involved in recipe development featured in magazines such as *Homemaker's, Cooking Light, Gardening Life* and more. She also contributes her nutritional analysis expertise to magazines such a *Wish* and *Canadian Family*. Amy's first cookbook, *Fiber Boost: Everyday Cooking for a Long Healthy Life*, was published by Key Porter in 2004. Eager to share her knowledge of healthy eating with the public, Amy also finds opportunities to speak to professional and community groups about how food trends are affecting the health of the North American population. Amy's team of researchers for this menu plan included Melanie Chislett and Shirley Walsh. All three worked hard to create an approachable yet appealing menu plan designed to help train you to develop better eating habits, making it easy for you to keep your health goals.

SECRETS TO SUCCESS— THE ANSWER LIES WITHIN

Everyone wants to be successful—at work, at home, in life. For every person or organization, success is interpreted differently. However "success" is defined, it most certainly involves the maximum fulfillment of potential that comes from reaching one's emotional quotient. With a wealth of practical experience and a gift for inspiring others, Dr. Reisner provides the raw tools necessary for goal achievement—whatever the goal may be. She teaches effective, present-day strategies for problem-solving, relating to colleagues, improving performance, reducing stress, and enhancing one's whole self. Specifically…

• adopting behavior that maximizes performance;

• avoiding behavior which can sabotage an individual's and, ultimately, an organization's productivity;

• focusing on what can, rather than what cannot, be changed.

Her didactic style is filled with humorous workplace anecdotes and resonates with virtually every audience—from board directors to salespeople to line employees. No matter how large the audience, Dr. Reisner's seminars are as accessible and beneficial for each individual as a one on one session in her Los Angeles psychiatric practice.

Her audiences include:

• Fortune 500 executives

• Mid-level professionals and trainees

• Entrepreneurs/small business owners

• Salespeople

• Investment bankers and management consultants

• Stockbrokers

• Attorneys

• Hospital administrators

• Professional organizations

• University faculty

CHAPTER 2

WHAT YOU WAITING FOR?

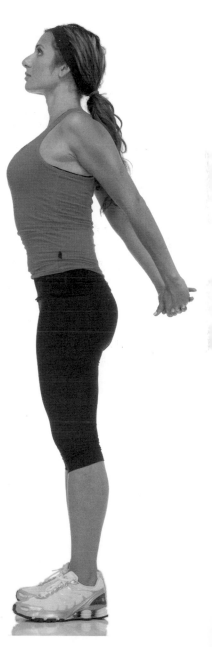

IMAGINE YOUR LIFE AS ONE LONG WALK DOWN that proverbial red carpet to a charmed winner's circle where all your goals, dreams, and aspirations have been realized. The question is how do you plan to get there, and achieve the chart-topping success you want and deserve? It literally starts with you, the way you feel about yourself deep down inside, and how you manifest that feeling to the world.

Nowhere is this more apparent than in your level of fitness, which is not only a signifier of your health and wellness, but also, I believe, of your all-round happiness. Your level of fitness says it all. It tells the world whether or not you are balanced; whether or not you want to live your life with all the energy and drive that you can physically and mentally exert, and whether or not you have made the effort to maximize your assets and commit to yourself. Everybody knows what his or her personal best is, and if you are not there or anywhere near it in terms of looking and feeling the way you want to, you have to ask yourself what you are waiting for.

My feeling is that if you have gone to the trouble of buying this book, your level of fitness is not where you want it or need it to be. The good news is that by buying this book, you are proving to yourself that you are motivated enough to do something about it. Just as I am sick and tired of women being made to feel bad about their bodies, you are probably sick and tired of tormenting yourself with those oh-so familiar recriminations. You know, those thoughts that run on a loop: I am overweight, so I am a loser. I pollute my body with junk food so I must be a loser. And I am definitely a loser because lately my idea of exercise has been lifting a few cold ones. Yes, those thoughts that probably alternate with the "I hate my body because it does not look like the girls in the Victoria Secrets show."

This mental Molotov cocktail of self-loathing and negativity could not be a more dangerous brew. "We believe it, but we are also validating it through messages from the outside," Dr. Reisner tells me. In other words, one crazy theory—"I should hate myself because I gained 10 pounds and did not lose it yesterday"—strengthens the other—"Heidi Klum is perfect and I am not."

The self-deprivation diets (more on that later) and the running-on-empty workout binges that cannot be maintained lead to the shame of failure. With this mental baggage bearing down so heavily on your psyche, is it any wonder that you find it impossible to get up off the couch? But you will, and you are going to.

The point is that however much you starve yourself or berate yourself for being "fat" while bemoaning the fact you were not blessed with Keira Knightley's or Sienna Miller's waif-like metabolism, it will not change the fact that you are who *you* are and look the way *you* look. Once you accept that, you will stop wasting time by wishing for the impossible and instead focus on all the possibilities that come with being the best possible you. As John Mayer would put it, your "body is a wonderland." It is only when you accept your innate shape in all its glory, and then commit to making it the best it can be, that your true Rock Star potential can be unleashed.

BELIEVE IT, ACHIEVE IT!

Conversely, if you do not believe it, you cannot and will not achieve it. In the first century there was a saying: "You are what you think," and the ancient philosophers said that we are not disturbed by things but how we perceive them, so it is our mindset that determines how we feel, act, and behave. As Dr. Reisner explains, "I wish I had a dollar for every client that came to me and said, 'You know what, Leslie? I've tried 25 times and, you know, I just don't believe it myself." It's a vicious cycle since the track record is that you have never been able to do it, so you will never be able to do it. And the feeling is that you are just not worth it. Dr. Reisner continues: "I always tell my patients in that situation that the best predictor of success in anything is the ability to visualize yourself being successful. If you go into it saying that I've tried to quit smoking 30 times and I've never been successful, that becomes your vision of yourself." And all too often this is a self-fulfilling prophesy, not just for smoking but for binge eating, negative obsessing, and all the other destructive behaviors that undermine your motivation to, say, hit the treadmill.

The bottom line is that your mind is your most powerful muscle, and motivation will come only after you have developed and executed a plan to flex it. You have to get past the deceptive comfort zone of the undermining interior dialogue, and realize that dwelling on negative experiences like failed diets and busting-at-the-seams jeans is just another way of avoidance. Really commit to this because it is truly fundamental: Your lasting physical evolution will come only through this mental revolution. Here's how to make it happen.

1. Stop Right There

And thank you very much, as the Spice Girls would finish the thought. You will definitely thank yourself if you change the negativity habit. I have always believed that the definition of insanity is repeating the same behavior over and over, and expecting a different result. This is also a sure path to failure. The only way to success is to change your behavior. According to Dr. Reisner, it takes months to break a habit, and it turns out that the best way to change a habit is to repeatedly do something different, and make that your habit instead. So every day for the next few months, I want you to stand in front of the mirror after you shower and really look at your body. Then make a choice not to make a negative statement. In fact, try something positive and see just how great that makes you feel. It will help if you think of yourself as your own best friend. You would never be verbally and mentally abusive to a friend, but rather, you would be supportive and encouraging. So why not do the same for yourself?

Now, I am not saying that you should not be realistic. If your thighs really are too big and you would like to lose weight, then acknowledge that, but do so without falling into the pattern of hateful, judgmental dialogue with yourself. Understand that some degree of judgment is necessary for change, but you have to make a distinction between the judgment of the situation and judgment of the person. In other words, judge the sin, not the sinner. "When people start demeaning themselves with derogatory statements, what usually results is anxiety and depression," explains Dr. Reisner, "and when people are anxious and depressed, they are far less likely to stay motivated and focused on the goal." It's simply counterproductive, so just cease and desist.

And if all else fails, paparazzi yourself. I am sure that David Hasselhoff will think twice before getting inebriated since a disturbing video of him wrestling a hamburger to the ground while losing control of his faculties surfaced on TMZ. "I do this with alcoholic patients," says Dr. Reisner. She advises that you tape yourself when you are taking out your frustrations on yourself, so that you can hear exactly what you sound like. A cautionary note: This will be difficult to hear without what Dr. Reisner calls punitive self-judgment. Don't go there!

2. Get Your Mojo Working

A mojo is an object believed to have magical powers, especially the power to keep evil spirits away. In blues music, which was the precursor to rock 'n' roll, legend Muddy Water, in his classic "I've Got My Mojo Working," often invoked it. As I believe there is nothing more powerful than words, make them your mojo. The minute that little voice in your head begins the negative train of thoughts like the ones I mentioned earlier, replace it with a mojo-boosting mantra. A mantra, by the way, is a word or phrase repeated during meditation to facilitate spiritual power and transformation of consciousness.

My mojo-boosting mantra is "Believe it, achieve it." Nothing motivates me quite like that phrase and I repeat it over in my mind countless times a day. You may have noticed that I have already mentioned it twice in this book. You can adopt it or, better yet, come up with an original phrase that turns on a similar switch in you. To give you some ideas, I have listed some relevant quotes from two motivational gurus who are considered Rock Stars in the self-help field and have been of great inspiration to me.

From Wayne Dyer:

- Be miserable. Or motivate yourself. Whatever has to be done, it's always your choice.

- Anything you really want, you can attain, if you really go after it.

- Deficiency motivation doesn't work. It will lead to a life-long pursuit of "try to fix me." Learn to appreciate what you have and where and who you are.

From Dale Carnegie:

- Develop success from failures. Discouragement and failure are two of the surest stepping stones to success.

- Feeling sorry for yourself, and your present condition, is not only a waste of energy but the worst habit you could possibly have.

- Inaction breeds doubt and fear. Action breeds confidence and courage. If you want to conquer fear, do not sit home and think about it. Go out and get busy.

And if not a mantra, a theme song may work for you. Songs whose lyrics propose an empowering message of self-love and acceptance should do the trick. Load songs such as Kanye West's "Everything I'm Not Makes Me Everything I Am" and Christina Aguilera's "I Am Beautiful" onto your iPod, press play, and imagine what you can achieve.

3. Don't Bring Sexy Back

In terms of body image, we as women have been habituated. This means that we have become so comfortable seeing the same thing over and over again—in this case, ultra-thin Hollywood bodies—that it becomes normal in our eyes. To compound the issue, women's bodies have been

---

JENNIFER'S EXTENDED MOTIVATIONAL PLAY LIST

The "Rocky" theme, a true classic, always inspires me to go for it and reach deep, even when I don't feel like it. Here are other Rock Star-worthy hits guaranteed to get your mind right from some of my favorite Rock Stars:

- Bob Sinclair: "Hold On"
- Cheryl Lynn: "Got to Be Real"
- Eminem: "Lose Yourself"
- Foo Fighters: "Learning to Fly"
- Garbage: "Push It"
- Gwen Stefani: "What You Waiting For?"
- Irene Cara: "What a Feeling"
- Kanye West: "Stronger"
- Moby: "Body Rock"
- Rupaul: "Supermodel"
- Stevie Nicks: "Stand Back"
- Survivor: "Eye of a Tiger"

objectified for decades, making us value them only as objects of desire. "A really neat visualization exercise I recommend for people who chronically judge and obsess over their bodies," says Dr. Reisner, "is to have them instead focus on its utility rather than just its cosmetics." In other words, you are likely to fall into a disheartening slump over a couple of cellulite dimples that your guy may glimpse as you slide out of bed backwards.

4. Justify Your Love

It makes it more difficult to criticize your body if you are nurturing that body. In her practice, Dr. Reisner has noticed that women who work out, drink water, and eat well may not be perfect, but the act of taking care of themselves sends the message that this body deserves it, and is therefore worth it. This puts them in better mental position to achieve their goals. It is important to acknowledge that your body has been good to you, and reward it by being kinder to it. Whether it is using a foot bath after a long day, indulging in a massage, or just making the healthy choice when a choice is to be made, the act of nurturing will allow you to avoid the Catch-22 situation. If you don't treat your body well, it won't be the body you want, and then you become self-doubting. Then once you become self-doubting, the nurturing stops. It is all about breaking that cycle, so why let it begin?

5. List Your Top 10

Despite your best intentions and efforts, there will be times when you are vulnerable to temptation. You may have had a tipsy night out with friends and find yourself at the burger drive-through at three a.m., Paris style. Or you may just be having a bad day and you automatically reach for something that you think will make you feel better. It won't, and you know that deep down inside, but at that moment your desire for that pizza, cookie, or tub of ice cream obliterates any thought of your goals. Says Dr. Reisner: "What I have my patients do all the time is to make a little card for their wallet. And on one side of the card I have them write down all the reasons why they want to achieve their goals, and on the flip side some of the obstacles they are going to face. So whenever they feel challenged, they have a reminder, a cue." This intervening process allows the mind to jump to the goals instead staying fixated on the taste you are going to experience, and thus instigate some control. You may want to cheat or even binge and you may even end up doing so, but once you've written and read the top 10 reasons why you want to stay fit, active, and healthy, it's a lot harder to screw up. It reminds you of your commitment to yourself. And it's all about you.

Let's Get Physical

Now that we have worked on the mind, and I think we can all agree that my mind games will be a lot more fun than yours, let's turn to your body. While your mental work focuses on motivation, this section is dedicated to realistic goal setting. You are who you are, and one of the quickest ways to get demotivated, not to mention crazed with frustration, is to aspire to the impossible by attempting to turn your body into something it is not supposed to be.

It reminds me of the story, perhaps apocryphal, about a top celebrity hair colorist—who shall remain nameless—and a certain mega-selling songbird client, who shall also remain nameless. The curly-haired, olive-skinned brunette wanted hair just like Gywneth Paltrow's. Aghast, the colorist explained that Gywneth, being a natural dirty blonde, was already halfway there, but still had to have a double process to get to a shade as light as her current one. Plus, Gywneth has the skin tone to carry it off. The colorist also advised the singer that if she went that light and that straight, it would not only literally destroy her hair, but the color would fail to flatter. But the diva insisted and the rest, as they say, was a series of god-awfully bad hair days until it all broke off close to the root. Thank God for wigs and extensions, and her fans were none the wiser.

I share this to point out that we as women abuse our hair as much as we abuse our bodies, but for some reason we tend to understand our hair mistakes. We've all had that one super-ugly perm in high school or that idiotic dye job in college, but we'd never do it again! At some point we all seem to decide that it is easier to work with the hair type that we were given, and realize that this is always the most attractive option. You may improve on nature, but you essentially just accept that this is it and get on with your life. Unfortunately, when it comes to our bodies, the obsession to compare and then change ourselves is so deeply ingrained that we will repeat the outlandish behavior ad infinitum. Saran Wrap in the sauna before a big event, anyone? Or have you, like Naomi

Campbell and Beyoncé, tried the Master Cleanse, which is essentially a 14-day water diet, with cayenne pepper and lemon juice as the only nutrients?

Now Beyoncé did the Master Cleanse in order to lose 20 pounds, which she did for her role in *Dreamgirls*, in which she played the sleek, stylish Deena. This was a character loosely based on Diana Ross during the period in which she clawed her way to the top of the 1960s super group, The Supremes. (Ironically, Beyoncé's wonderful performance was overshadowed by the Oscar-winning role of the very zaftig Jennifer Hudson, whose character, Effie, was ousted from the girl group because—drum roll—she was too fat.) There were several press reports about Beyonce's new figure, but I missed Bootylicious Beyoncé. And so did Beyonce. After filming she announced that she was having a great time regaining her curves and is now as filled out as she ever was. Skinny Beyoncé reminded me of that friend we all have—the voluptuous one who, though she has managed to get herself down to her mythical ideal weight, she somehow doesn't look as good as she did before. For that person, as the old funk classic says, there is just more bounce to the ounce!

Science proposes a theory that seemingly backs this up. It holds that each person may possess an inherent "set point" weight, which the brain attempts to maintain, and that this set point may vary for each individual depending on a variety of factors that include nature (genetic disposition) and nurture (like your environment, for instance). Although this suggests that the set point may be changed with diet and exercise, essentially each person may be predisposed to naturally maintaining a specific body weight. Therefore, if you maintain a healthy lifestyle that includes proper nutrition and regular fitness, the body will naturally settle at the size it is meant to be.

There is a saying gaining popularity among the single set—"Perfect size for me." The idea is that everyone has an ideal potential hook-up, which may be outside the parameters of what is considered normal, acceptable, or perfect. Keep the meaning but switch its focus. Whether you want to lose weight, gain muscle, or both, there's an ideal potential you and that is your goal in a nutshell—to be the perfect size for you.

TYPE A LIST

Starlets complain that Hollywood is rife with type-casting, but in this case it is a good thing. When it comes to our bodies, biology and genetics have assigned each of us one of three types. We all fit (pun intended) into one of three body types—endomorph, ectomorph, or mesomorph—that determines what our basic physique is, whatever shape we happen to be in. And, yes, some of these shapes are smaller than others, but it doesn't necessarily make it better or more enticing. Think of Jessica Biel, a normal-size woman, who is positively Herculean by Hollywood's standards, yet she has buffed up her body into the Sexiest Woman Alive category, according to *Esquire* magazine, and replaced the model-like Cameron Diaz in the affections of one Justin Timberlake. And even a beauty, celebrated for her body, is not immune. "I want to be a big, fleshy voluptuous woman with curves. I want a big bum, but I don't have one," Cameron Diaz has said. So go figure, and while we do, can we all just get happy with ourselves?

Knowledge is power, so I am asking you to identify your body type to better adjust your goals and expect results to your reality. Remember, one body type is not better than the other, which is why I have included examples of Rock Stars who fit into each type and who all look ridiculously hot when they are in optimum shape.

- You are an endomorph if you have a curvaceous body with relatively large bones. Your hips are wider than your shoulders and you tend to carry your weight below your waist.
- *Rock Star endomorphs:* Alicia Keyes, Jennifer Lopez, Janet Jackson, Kelly Clarkson, Beyoncé, Mary J. Blige.

Your theme song: Beyoncé's "Bootylicious" for the same reasons that Kanye West once rapped, "nobody likes a small tight ass." However Sir Mix-a-lot's "Baby Got Back" will do in a pinch.

- You are an ectomorph if you are slender with a small to medium frame. Your hips and shoulders are in proportion with each other and you tend to be a bit angular.
- *Rock Star ectomorphs:* Posh Spice (despite her two new girls), Christina Aguilera (despite hers as well), Sheryl Crow, Joss Stone, Whitney Houston, Celine Dion.
- *Your theme song:* "Girls on Film" by Duran Duran, as ectomorphs tend to be those natural size 0s who become models if they are tall enough and, if shorter, have the body type currently coveted in Hollywood. (Just remember: At one point, so was Marilyn Monroe, who was a very large size 8 at her thinnest!)

- You are a mesomorph if you are athletic with a fairly muscular build. You tend to be rectangular with your weight balanced on your body, although your shoulders tend to be broader than your hips.
- *Rock Star mesomorphs:* Gwen Stefani, Britney Spears, Jessica Simpson, Madonna, Carrie Underwood, Mariah Carey.
- *Your theme song:* "Brick House" by The Commodores, who believe that you are "mighty, mighty" and "the only one built like an amazon." Lionel and the guys also believe that your strong shape is "everything a woman needs to get a man."

With that said, know that these types are a guide, and many of you may not be strictly just one or the other. You may be an endomorph with a mesomorph's ability to build muscle, an ectomorph with curves, or an endomorph with a little less on top.

Either way, it's all good and about to get Rock Star better. As you follow this program, you will come to know and understand your body in a way that you never have before, and you will also come to realize that there is no better judge of what it is than you!

WEIGHTY MATTERS

Aaliyah sang "age ain't nothing but a number," but I have to say the same thing about weight. People get hung up on the number, but as we just learned, there are several different types of bodies, and a long, lithe temptress of 5-foot 10-inches tall and a curvy, voluptuous cutie of 5-foot 4-inches tall can both weigh 130 pounds and still be healthy and fit. What's more important is whether that 130 pounds consists of "I have Pizza Pizza on speed dial" body fat or "I always hit the gym" muscle.

It is always good to have a target and a scale, which is useful in tracking progress. However, many women begin to weigh compulsively when trying to lose weight, and get discouraged when the weight loss is not immediate and dramatic. Since I recommend losing at a slow and steady space, track your progress by weighing every 14 days. Do it after your menstrual cycle is complete to avoid skewed results due to hormonal bloating, and first thing in the morning after you relieve yourself and before you eat. Also try to avoid meals high in salt and any alcohol the night before as they lead to water retention. Weigh yourself while naked using the same scale every time, as they can vary in calibration, for consistency.

Now, in an attempt to quell any reason for obsessive behavior, some trainers I know advise their clients to avoid the scale completely and track their progress by the fit of their clothes. I don't particularly like this method because stretch fabric in women's clothing has become very common and they essentially shrink to fit. Also, many of us wear jeans 24/7, and we all know that the more you wear them, the looser they get. So, of course, if you lose a large amount of weight, the difference will be apparent in the look and feel of your clothes, but for the more incremental stages, stick to the scale.

Many of us get obsessed with having a low number, which not only seems to connote thinness, but is also perceived as being more feminine. The truth is that getting toned means increased muscle, and muscle weighs more than fat. With increased muscle, you will look leaner, trimmer, and thinner, but you just may weigh more.

The Tale of the Tape

And while we're at it, let's not forget that you can pinch an inch. Much like the scale, the tape measure will help you stay on track. Measure yourself when you weigh, and under the same conditions. When you are taking the measurements, do not pull the tape too snugly—it should not be a squeeze, nor should the tape measure dig into your skin. Also, do not manipulate your body by flexing, tensing, or breathing in or out as it will distort the measurements. Measure your bust (at the nipple line); your chest (right under your bust); each arm (at the widest circumference of the upper area between your shoulder and elbow); your waist (at its smallest part); your hips (at the widest part when your feet are together); each thigh (at the largest area); and each calf (at the widest point).

So weighing and measuring may give you the numbers as you start walking this Rock Star way, but you need a more targeted analysis to see how your weight and body composition stacks up with your health. For that you need to calculate your body mass index, or BMI, and your body fat percentage. Here's how:

Body Mass Index

BMI is a calculation based on a person's height and weight. The result indicates if a person is underweight, "normal" weight for them, overweight, or obese. According to the Canadian Guidelines for Healthy Weight, "The BMI is widely accepted as a simple and fairly accurate way to assess body weight in relation to health for most people between 20 and 65 years of age."

Please keep in mind that the BMI is only a guide and is not perfect. It doesn't consider individual factors such as bone and muscle mass. For instance, if you are of small stature, your BMI may read unhealthily low, and if you are muscular, your BMI may read unhealthily high when in fact you are healthy.

To calculate your BMI, divide your weight (in pounds) by your height (in inches), then divide that result by your height (in inches again), and then multiply that result by 703.

So if your BMI is under 20, it does not indicate a health risk if you are genetically small. However, your low body weight is a health risk if it is achieved and maintained through chronic dieting and food restriction because the chances of morbidity (the presence of illness and disease) and mortality are greatly increased. A severely low BMI could also result in certain types of cancer, infertility, anemia, nutrient deficiencies, the suppression of menstruation, infertility, electrolyte imbalances, dehydration, constipation, bloating, and psychological issues.

If your BMI is between 20–25, you are at what is considered a healthy weight for most people.

If your BMI is between 25–27, and you are not an extremely muscled person or an athlete, then you are considered overweight and may suffer related health problems.

If your BMI is over 27, your chances of mortality are also sharply increased with a host of serious health problems coming into play. They include infertility and high-risk pregnancies, coronary heart disease, hypertension, diabetes, cancers of the breast and the endometrium, gallstones, osteoarthritis of the knee, sleep disorders, stress incontinence, and psychosocial problems.

If your BMI is under 20 due to an eating disorder, or over 25 due to obesity, you should seek medical advice before embarking on No Gym Required.

Body Fat Percentage

Your body fat percentage is probably the most important number of them all because it is a precise measure of your body composition in a way the BMI is not. A high ratio of body fat, as opposed to lean body mass (which consists of your bones, muscles, and organs), can promote premature aging and a host of serious medical conditions from heart disease and high blood pressure to diabetes and cancer.

The two most accurate ways to measure your proportion of fat are either a DEXA scan (a type of X-ray that measures both bone density and soft tissue mass) and hydrostatic or underwater weighing, which calculates the fat percentage based on your body density determined by the amount of water you displaced. As these methods are not widely available, two alternative methods practised at most gyms and health clubs through certified physical trainers should do the trick.

The skin-fold caliper test measures the thickness of fatty tissue by pinching a fold of skin at several specific points on the body—sometimes as little as three or as much as seven places—which are then calculated using a formula that estimates the body fat percentage.

The body-fat scale uses bioelectrical impedance. A low-level electrical current runs through the body, and the more resistance there is to the current, the larger the percentage of fat. However, the results are influenced by outside factors, so step on the body-fat scale first thing in the morning only after you have relieved yourself and before you have eaten. Drink a small bottle of water, as hydration is necessary for a proper reading to take place.

Here are the recommended body-fat percentage guidelines. If your essential fat percentage is below the recommended number or if your percentage is in the obesity range, you should seek medical advice before embarking on No Gym Required.

Ages	Males	Females
20–29	10–15%	18–22%
30–39	12–16%	20–24%
40–49	14–18%	21–25%
50+	15–19%	22–26%
Athletes	5–8%	12–18%
Essential fat	3%	12%
Obesity	25+%	32+%

Metabolism and Muscle

Thanks to Van Halen and their infamous demand that all brown M&Ms be banished from their backstage area, these candies have become the ultimate punch line in Rock Star diva behavior. But the

M&Ms that will matter most to you divas-in-the-making are metabolism and muscle, and how they work together. Metabolism is the rate at which the body burns calories while performing the complex chemical interactions that provide energy and nutrients to sustain life. In other words, the amount of calories you burn by just being alive. So your individual or resting metabolic rate can be high, which allows you to easily maintain your target size and lose weight. Actor Ellen Pompeo describes herself as a true waif who has trouble keeping weight on. Or, like Oprah Winfrey, your metabolism may be low, which makes it more difficult to keep the weight off. (In fact, Oprah's sluggish metabolism has been traced to a thyroid problem. More on that later.) And although your metabolic rate is genetically determined and declines with age, building muscle mass is one way to boost it. The more muscle you have, the higher your metabolism, as it has been said that each pound of muscle burns an extra 50 calories a day, while each pound of fat burns approximately 2 calories a day. So the goal, when losing weight, is to keep your metabolism up by getting rid of fat while increasing muscle mass. This is how you will maintain a healthy body composition. And while you're at it, increasing your aerobic exercise, as well as simply being more active throughout the day, will help. Dieting alone will cause you to lose muscle along with fat, so it is imperative to do exercise that builds muscle three or four times a week. Again, if your goal is to look and be smaller, adding muscle is what will actually do the trick as fat takes up three times the volume of muscle.

Resting Metabolic Rates (RMRs) differ from individual to individual depending on age, genetics, gender, body mass, body composition, and level of fitness, which is why it is possible to boost it. Here is how to figure out yours using the Harris-Benedict equation. To convert pounds to kilograms, multiply the number of pounds by 0.4535923744953.

For women, the resting metabolic rate = 655.1 + (9.563 × weight in kilograms) + 1.850 × height in centimeters) - (4.676 × age).

For men, the resting metabolic rate = 66 + (13.7 × weight in kilograms) + (5 × height in centimeters) - (6.8 × age in years).

Now hang on to your number as it will be important in the next chapter.

CHAPTER 3

THE GREATEST LOVE OF ALL

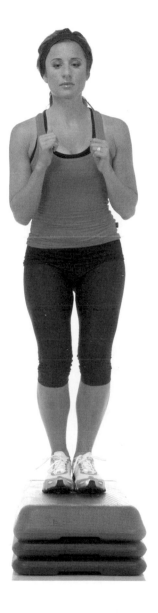

I ADMIT IT, I AM OBSESSED WITH FOOD AND I love to eat. It is my greatest love. But I absolutely hate diets. Diets are the devil! Extreme and restrictive, they play havoc with your health (leading to anything from hair loss to heart trouble) and are impossible to maintain for any length of time. And then when you go off, say, the Watercress Diet or the All-the-Protein-You-Can-Eat Diet and just eat normally, biology dictates that you will regain the weight with some more to spare. Psychology also dictates that you will probably binge. Why go to such weird lengths when it is really quite simple? Diet is the foundation of any healthy fitness program—it's 70 percent of the battle. If you have more input (what you eat) versus output (what you burn off), you will gain weight and not lose it. That is, you can work out all day, but if you eat more calories than you burn, then the equation adds up to weight gain. The key is to find an effective, goal-oriented system of eating that is realistic and can become a regular part of your life. And when I suggest something for your diet, this is what I mean: the dictionary definition as in the food, drink, and nutrients that one consumes, not the nonsense out there.

ALL ABOARD THE CRAZY TRAIN

What not to do and what not to think, brought to you by some of your favorite celebrities.

Sara Ramirez:
I basically starved myself [when trying to break into television], living on a stick of celery, some peanut butter, and two protein shakes a day, and worked out like a fiend. Sure enough, I lost 25 pounds and booked a TV pilot—scary because it was almost like a reward for treating myself in an unhealthy way.

Liv Tyler:
I've been working since I was 14, and [being pregnant] was the first time in my life I wasn't on a diet and didn't have that kind of pressure.

Elizabeth Hurley:
I have to squeeze myself into quite a few bikinis. It's definitely a part of my job … not to be too fat.

Kim Cattrall:
I diet every day of my life. It's part of my discipline.

Anne Hathaway:
I basically stuck with fruit, vegetables, and fish [to slim down for *The Devil Wears Prada*]. I wouldn't recommend that. Emily Blunt and I would clutch each other and cry because we were so hungry.

Marcia Cross:
I have often felt there was a lot of pressure on me to look good…. It's like they pay me not to eat. It's a living hell.

Gwen Stefani:
I've always been on a diet, ever since I was in the sixth grade. It's an ongoing battle and it's a nightmare. I feel like if I don't eat, I might lose one more pound.

Carrie Underwood:
I'm slightly obsessive-compulsive about what I eat, more than I should be.

Carmen Electra:
I tried the not-eating anorexic thing, the anorexic diet, and for me it didn't work. I would feel like I was going to pass out.

Hilary Duff:
There was definitely a time … when I was pretty obsessed with my body and my weight, but I'm better not stressing about my body all the time…. You lose some happiness when that's all you think about.

Linda Evangelista:
I don't diet. I just don't eat as much as I want to.

Salma Hayek:
I refuse to become part of this perfect-body syndrome. I like my body. It looks good on-screen, and it's not because it's perfect. I accept it and wear it like a good dress…. One guy I dated said, "You're beautiful, but you're soft. You can't compete with other actresses in Hollywood because everyone's in shape and working out." I said, "Very nice to meet you. Goodbye!"

Now before we get started, I want you to delve a little deeper into the relationship between you and food. Keep a food diary for seven days as it will take you through the work week and the weekend, therefore covering the entire spectrum of your everyday life. Eat as you normally would and write down every last morsel you put in your mouth. Also record the time you ate it at and exactly how you were feeling when you did so. After the seven days, review your journal and make a note of what triggered your cravings. If you found that you reached for some mac and cheese every other night at 10 p.m., there's probably an emotional or psychological trigger for that. Remember what I told you in Chapter 1: Change the habit. Take a bubble bath or walk round the block instead. Now if you wanted and indulged in a chocolate bar every afternoon at 3 p.m., there is quite possibly a chemical reason for the craving and a nutritional way to offset it. Knowledge is power and control.

So instead of hotel rooms, we Rock Stars are trashing diets. Instead of trying to follow these impossible gimmicks, we are going back to basics using the most effective nutritional methods. Follow the Rock Star food principles to subdue cravings, boost your metabolism, promote health and wellness (and therefore beauty), and still have leeway for a little fun. Cheat day anyone?

PRINCIPLE 1: GET FRESH, GO WILD: EAT NATURAL AND ORGANIC

Eat natural and organic foods always. This is fundamental to health and therefore fitness, and I cannot stress enough how important this is. Processed foods and those with preservatives are laden with hidden sugars and fats, many unknown to nature. Even meats and so-called natural produce like fruits and vegetables are filled with antibiotics and pesticides, which are proven toxins. Your body's food-processing mechanism is just not designed to handle them. Have you noticed the proliferation of health problems from weird new allergies to rampant obesity and the hormonal-related cancers in women that are just a generation old? These new materials are adversely affecting our bodies, and we keep poisoning ourselves with them because we have come to believe they are normal. They are not meant to enter our bodies, and when they do, they sit in our system and clog it up with junk. They not only have no redeeming qualities, but, worse yet, they make us sick and fat.

This is why I follow this "fresh from the ground up" principle. My preference is for things grown in the ground and that subsist close to land, whether that's fresh vegetables and fruit, grass-fed beef, wild (not farmed) fish, or free-range chicken. And opt for organic whenever possible. Yes, it's more expensive, but I think we Rock Stars know that our health is worth the investment. And this is a commandment: Know thy food sources whenever possible. Eating locally and seasonally is always your best bet for your health and for the environment. You know exactly where the produce is coming from and it has not spent days on a truck and in a warehouse before reaching your table! For maximum nutrients, fresh fruits and veggies should be eaten within three or four days of being picked. Your carbon footprint will be reduced, and it's also more fun and keeps you in touch with nature. I like shopping at markets where selection of the season's bounty is plentiful. It's an immediate natural food rush. And one of my favorite summer pastimes is to go pea-picking—they're sweet, tasty, low-fat, and low-cal. Some people like to go apple-picking. You should try it. Apples are one of my all-time greatest hit foods, but more on that later.

When you shop in the grocery store, stay on the perimeter where the fresh produce, meat, fish, and dairy aisles are. Avoid the middle aisles, which are stacked with processed foods that might be labeled as "healthy" or "low-fat" or "low-carb," but in fact often have ingredients used to give them longer shelf life, but are unhealthy. There will be more on that later too. Dubbed so-called "convenience" foods, these products can wreak havoc on your system and make it hard to meet your weight-loss goals. On the other hand, breaking down foods that are natural and unprocessed not only boosts your health and wellness but also burns calories!

WHAT IS ORGANIC

Organic food is produced by farmers who use renewable resources and the conservation of soil and water to preserve the environment. Organic meat, poultry, eggs, and dairy products come from animals that are not given antibiotics or growth hormones. Organic food is produced without using most conventional pesticides, fertilizers made with synthetic ingredients or sewage sludge, and bioengineering or ionizing radiation. Before a product can be labeled "organic," a government-approved certifier inspects the farm where the food is grown to make sure the farmer is following all the rules necessary to meet organic standards. Companies that handle or process organic food before it gets to your local supermarket or restaurant must be certified, too. Food labeled organic must be at least 95 percent organic.

—The National Organic Program/USDA

SO FRESH, SO CLEAN

Clean protein is a must if you want to prevent disease, premature aging, and get and stay in shape. Rock Stars demand and deserve the best, so choose the following:

- *Wild fish versus farmed fish:* Relatively low in calories and saturated fat as well as a great source of vitamins, minerals, and essential fatty acids, it is tempting to have fish in your diet every day, but please do not do so if you are eating farmed fish. Unfortunately, most of the fish found in grocery stores are farmed. This is bad news because the conditions that fish are farmed in leaves them full of toxic methylmercury, PCBs (artificial chemicals used in electrical transformers and gas pipelines), as well as viruses and bacteria. This cancels out the nutritional value, doesn't it? Always, always, always request fresh wild fish. And even without the toxicity, remember this: Farmed salmon are fattier than wild salmon because they are fed so much more meal and oil. For more information and to advocate for healthier and more sustainable fish, log on to www.seafoodchoices.com, the Web site of the Seafood Choices Alliance. Also look for environmentally friendly brands. I like RainCoast, a brand of a sustainable fish cannery. They ensure that their products are wild and are tested to ensure that they are low in mercury.

- *Grass-fed beef versus feed-lot beef:* I know that some of you who may be reading this may be vegetarians, but I have to be honest in telling you that meat is a great diet food. It builds muscle, stimulates the metabolism, and is packed with iron, which is important for us women—that is, if it doesn't contain the harmful antibiotics, steroids, and hormones. Cows (as are lambs and goats) are designed to eat and digest grass, which they can easily convert into protein and fat. In feed-lot beef, which is readily available today, cows are fed grain because it is cheaper to do as it fattens them up faster. This is the problem: Cows are unable to digest grain on their own and must be pumped full of antibiotics in order to do so. It also profoundly disturbs their digestion, which weakens their immune systems and leads to liver problems, among under things. More disturbingly, it creates an acidic stomach environment similar to ours, which makes us more vulnerable to infection from viruses like E. coli. Do yourself and those poor cows a favor and switch to grass-fed beef. Not only is it just plain purer, it is lower in saturated fat and higher in omega-3 fatty acids (see the table of good fats and bad fats). Eat grass-fed beef and avoid the health concerns while getting all the amazing benefits of the high protein, which is imperative in building muscle and boosting metabolism. Double up with organic practices and you're golden.

WHAT'S YOUR BEEF

Another caveat with beef is that it is high in unhealthy fat. Get the benefits of beef and minimize the fat content:

1. Look for "loin" and "round" in the names of the cuts as these tend to be the leanest.

2. Marbling refers to the bits of fat that are scattered throughout a cut of beef. The marbling helps to make the meat tender and flavorful, but it will not significantly increase the level of fat that is consumed, especially if the beef is cooked using low-fat cooking methods and if the outer layers of fat are removed before cooking.

3. Low-fat cooking methods include broiling, grilling, steaming, stewing, braising, baking, and roasting.

4. When cooking beef in the oven, place the beef on a rack so that fat can drain off as it cooks.

5. Skim fat from the surface of beef soups, stews, and sauces before serving. Chill soups and stews because the fat will rise to the surface and can be removed in solid pieces.

- *Free-range chicken versus factory-farm chicken:* Free-range or pastured chicken and other poultry are raised outdoors and get a percentage of their food from natural foraging, along with grain. Not only is this more humane—we have all seen images of those small, stacked cages that chickens are bred in these days—but it is healthier. The chickens are not in the cramped quarters that cause disease to be easily spread, and it is less likely that antibiotics will be used. These chickens are also free of hormones (meant to fatten them up), as well as pesticides and herbicides. The choice is clear.

- *Protein for vegetarians:* Most plant proteins, with the exception of certain ones like soy, do not have all the amino acids that make them complete. Plant proteins are found in legumes, nuts, and whole grains. For meals, combine more than one plant protein source—that is, legumes with grains or nuts and seeds with legumes to make sure you get optimum nutrition.

PRINCIPLE 2: COUNT DOWN: EAT WITH CALORIES AND PORTION CONTROL IN MIND

Nothing is more basic than this: Take in less calories and exert more energy and I guarantee that you will lose weight. Take in more calories and exert less energy, and you'll gain. Duh! Now in the last chapter, we figured out how to calculate our resting metabolic rate. Here we will use that number to calculate precisely what your daily caloric intake should be. To do that, factor in your activity level:

If you are sedentary (little or no exercise): Calorie calculation = RMR × 1.2

If you are lightly active (light exercise/sports one to three days a week): Calorie calculation = RMR × 1.375

If you are moderately active (moderate exercise or sports three to five days a week): Calorie calculation = RMR × 1.55

If you are very active = RMR × 1.725 (hard exercise or sports six or seven days a week): Calorie calculation = RMR × 1.725

If you are extra active (very hard daily exercise or sports and a physical job or twice-daily training): Calorie calculation = RMR × 1.9

Now that you have your daily caloric requirement, here's what to do with it. To maintain your current weight, eat that amount of calories every day. If you need to gain weight, add 200–250 calories a day, and I don't mean junk calories from milkshakes and doughnuts but healthy protein and carbs. Also, muscle-building exercise will help. And if you want to lose weight, cut 500 calories a day and burn off 500 more with cardiovascular exercise to lose approximately 2 pounds per week.

Let us not forget portions. In this super-size me society, we have lost sight of what a normal serving size should really look like. Generally, a serving of meat is 4 ounces—it should be the size of a deck of cards. A serving of fruit and vegetables is a cup, with 2 cups for leafy green vegetables. A serving of rice, pasta, and other grains is about a half cup. There will be more on this later when we decode food labels, but check the serving size carefully. One bottle or one package isn't necessarily one serving, so you may be taking in twice the calories than you think you are.

PRINCIPLE 3: MORE, MORE, MORE: EAT TO BOOST YOUR METABOLISM

Instead of the traditional three square meals a day, eat five times a day at consistent four-hour intervals. Of those five times, three should be meals of 300–400 calories, and two of them should be healthy snacks. (See the

Personal Chef Rock Star Recipes and Jennifer's Rock Star Snack List below.) This way your metabolism is constantly fueled and burning. And always start with breakfast as this kick-starts everything. Never skip a meal as it will have exactly the opposite effect of what you intend. When the body is deprived of food, it goes into starvation mode by holding onto calories in order to conserve energy. You will then store fat instead of burning it, so eat up. And to amplify the effect, add the following:

Mega Metabolism Boosters

Thermogenesis is the production of heat in a person's body by either physiological or metabolic processes, and is a key component in boosting your metabolism. To do so, try the following:

- *Omega-3 and omega-6 essential fatty acids:* These are the two EFAs not created by the body itself. The omega-3s are found in cold-water fish such as salmon, mackerel, and herring; green leafy vegetables; seeds and nuts such as flaxseeds (and flax oil) and walnuts. The omega-6s are more common and found in animal fats, most cooking oils, margarine, and soy. Try to get them in your food, but I suggest backing that up by taking a supplement. Apart from the host of bodily systems these EFAs affect, such as maximizing nutrition and expelling toxic waste at a cellular level, they also regulate the thyroid hormones that keep the metabolism revved up . EFAs support both fat metabolism and carbohydrate metabolism—two excellent reasons to get enough of them.

- *Hot and spicy foods:* From jalapeno to chili to Scotch bonnet, pile on the pepper and don't cool it on the curry as this is one sure-fire way to stoke thermogenesis. This is also a great way to experiment and add another dimension to your life as many hot and spicy foods tend to be ethnic. Whether Indian, Ethiopian, or Jamaican, it sure beats another piece of pizza in the boredom stakes. And by the way, have you noticed that you eat a lot less when something is hot and spicy?

- *Green tea:* Learn to love this gift from the East. It contains high concentrations of catechin polyphenols, which intensify levels of fat oxidation by inhibiting the movement of sugar into fat cells, as well as thermogenesis. But green tea's benefits do not stop there. Apart from aiding heart health and indigestion, it will also help the skin look younger longer as it is full of antioxidants that fend off the free radicals that lead to cellular breakdown. Make green tea a constant—model Sophie Dahl claims she went from a size 16 to an 8 due to constantly sipping it. Throw a couple of green teabags in your water bottle and go.

TEA HOUSE

And don't stop at just green tea. Herbal teas on the whole are a clean, pure, and healthy way to hydrate, curb cravings, and satisfy an oral fixation. For a change of pace, brew up some of these not-so-typical teas.

- *White tea:* The silvery feathery leaves of white tea come from the same plant as green and black teas, but they're harvested earlier and have a more delicate, sweeter flavor. Research shows that it fights viruses and infections and may be even more powerful than green tea in protecting against cancer.

- *Ginseng tea:* Ginseng is a sure-fire fatigue fighter. The active ingredient, ginsenosides, works on the pituitary-adrenal axis, increasing resistance to stress while boosting metabolism and stamina. Ginseng also helps balance hormones and gives lasting energy all day.

- *Burdock tea:* Burdock (also known as gobo) is a root used in Japanese cooking and is a strong liver detoxifier and hormone-balancing herb. (The liver is the major calorie-burning organ and metabolizes fat.) Burdock contains a carbohydrate called inulin, which strengthens the liver. The tea is similar in flavor to asparagus when boiled and can be mixed with apple cider for an alternative to your regular salad dressing.

- *Nettle tea:* A fantastic source of potassium, calcium, and magnesium that can give you the energy you need to exercise. Nettle tea is a great kidney cleanser—the kidney detoxifies the body and keeps it chemically balanced. Nettle has a gentle, grassy flavor and, when infused overnight, it turns an intense emerald green.

PRINCIPLE 4: ALL TOGETHER NOW: EAT A BALANCED DIET

Now here's another back-to-basics idea that may seen novel in this age of banishing carbs or fats or whatever happens to be the demonized food group du jour. The fact is that the body needs all the food groups to get the full complement of nutrients it needs to function properly. Do not eliminate a food group; instead, the key is to balance the food groups and make sure that each food is the healthy choice in its category. Just as there is good music and bad music, there are good proteins and bad proteins, good fats and bad fats, as well as good carbs and bad carbs. I will explain it all as we progress through this eating section. Just make sure that the protein is lean and clean, and is at least half of the value of carbohydrates. The carbs should be slow-burning complex carbs such as fruits, vegetables, and fiber. And make sure that fats—the good kind—make up at least a quarter of your calories. It is necessary for health, beauty, and, believe it or not, weight loss.

Good Fats

Good fats can lower your risk of heart disease by reducing the total level of cholesterol and low-density lipoprotein (LDL) cholesterol in your blood.

- *Monounsaturated fats:* Avocados, most nuts, as well olive, peanut, and canola oils

- *Polyunsaturated fats:* Vegetable oils, such as safflower, corn, sunflower, soy, and cottonseed oils

Bad Fats

Bad fats can increase your risk of heart disease by increasing your total cholesterol level, including LDL ("bad") cholesterol,

- *Saturated fat and dietary cholesterol:* Meat, poultry, seafood, eggs, dairy and dairy products such as lard

---

THE SKINNY ON FAT

Not only is fat a key energy source, it is also a nutrient used in the production of cells as well as compounds that regulate blood pressure, heart rate, blood vessel constriction, blood clotting, and the nervous system. Dietary fat also carries fat-soluble vitamins—vitamins A, D, E, and K—from your food into your body. Fat also helps maintain healthy hair and skin, protects vital organs, keeps your body insulated, and provides a sense of fullness after meals. But high-fat foods are dense in calories and overindulging, as we all know, can lead to obesity. The key is to choose the right kinds of fats and eat even those in moderation (fat contains 9 calories a gram, compared with 4 calories per gram for protein and carbohydrates) and to stay away from the wrong kind.

We've already been through the benefits of EFAs, but now that we're talking good fats, it's worth stressing again just how important these essential fatty acids are.

and butter, as well as coconut, palm, and other tropical oils

Really, Really Bad Fat—The Absolute Worst!

- *Trans-fat acids:* Also referred to as trans-fatty acids, trans fat is created by adding hydrogen to vegetable oil through a process called hydrogenation in order to preserve packaged baked goods. It is used in shortenings, some margarines, crackers, cookies and cakes, as well as fried fast foods, such as doughnuts and french fries. And apart from its calorie-laden, artery-clogging, heart-stopping, obesity-promoting properties, trans fats are also thought to be carcinogenic as they promote oxidation at the cellular level. So, in other words, eat no evil!

Trans fats are considered such a health blight that there is a movement underway to rid restaurants and grocery shelves of them. The organization Ban Trans Fat's Campaign to Ban Partially Hydrogenated Oils (www.bantransfat.com) has sued Kraft to ban trans fats from Oreo cookies and, as a result, trans fats were removed from them and reduced or eliminated in 650 other Kraft products. The organization also successfully sued McDonald's to admit to its customers that it had not switched to a lower trans-fat cooking oil. As a result, McDonald's agreed to donate $7 million to the American Heart Association for a trans fat program. Fortunately, the need to banish trans fats has caught on among progressive health officials. The American Food and Drug Administration (FDA) has ordered that all packaged food must list trans fat content, while (as of this writing) regulations have been passed banning them in restaurants in New York, Philadelphia, and Toronto. But take matters into your own hands. Ban them from your life. You won't eat them if you don't buy them. And while you're at it, there are other ingredients you need to take out and not just out of your grocery cart.

BAD FAT-BUSTING TIPS

You will notice that some of these items, like beef, chicken, shellfish, eggs, and some dairy, are foods that I suggest you eat. This is not the contradiction that it would at first seem. The muscle-building and metabolism-boosting benefits of the protein in beef, chicken, and seafood far outweigh the issues of saturated fat and dietary cholesterol if you eat these foods in moderation and in the right way. I have already told you how to best minimize the fat in beef. Also remember to:

1. Eat chicken without the skin as most of the fat is stored right under it. And stick to chicken breasts, which are the leanest part of the bird.
2. With dairy, always go for the low- or non-fat versions.
3. Pass on the yolks, where the fat and cholesterol are stored, and use just the whites to make your morning scrambled eggs. If you must, just use one yolk for taste and color.

And though actually quite low in fat, shellfish, which are full of important vitamins, minerals, and, ironically, EFAs, have got a bad rap due to their dietary cholesterol content. However, studies have shown that dietary cholesterol does not necessarily turn into cholesterol in the body the way saturated fats do.

COMPARISON OF DIETARY FATS CHART				
DIETARY FAT	FATTY ACID CONTENT NORMALIZED TO 100 PERCENT			
	Saturated Fat	Mono-unsaturated Fat	Poly-unsaturated Fat	Linoleic Acid
Canola oil	7	61	11	21
Safflower oil	8	77	1	14
Flaxseed oil	9	16	57	18
Sunflower oil	12	16	1	71
Corn oil	15	75	1	9
Olive oil	15	75	1	*
Soybean oil	15	23	8	54
Peanut oil	19	48	*	33
Cottonseed oil	27	19	*	54
Lard	43	47	1	9
Palm oil	51	39	*	10
Butterfat	68	28	1	3
Coconut Oil	91	7	*	2

What's the point? There is none!!!

DYE

Of the seven commonly used in foods (Red 3, Red 40, Blue 1, Blue 2, Green 3, Yellow 5, Yellow 6) from bottled cherries to the coating of headache pills, four have been shown to cause cancer. Are we that detached from reality as a culture that we need strawberry jam to look redder than it actually is? Do we need to snack on bright orange artificialities when a tangerine will do and be a million times better for us? I've said it before, and I'll say it again: Just go natural.

Major yuck factor: Dyes are derived from artificial coal tar. Not only does it wreak havoc on the body, consider the ecosystem.

Redeeming quality: None

Remember: Like all great artists, you'll learn to love the colors found in nature.

REFINED GRAINS

Refined grains are anything but nutritious. Grains go from whole to refined when the bran (which is the fiber-rich outer layer) and the germ (which is the nutrient-rich inner part) are removed to make the grain easier to cook. So along with fiber, the folic acid, magnesium, and vitamins are also removed, leaving the food essentially stripped of all nutritional value and digestive ease. The white starches so prevalent in our diets (like bread, rice, and pasta) are refined as are most cereals. If you don't already eat whole grains like oatmeal, barley, rye, and brown rice, make the change. They lower cholesterol, reduce the risk of cancer, aid the absorption of nutrients and the elimination process, while keeping you safe from the evil of empty, fattening calories.

Major yuck factor: Who can forget that wheelbarrow of fat that Oprah brought out on her show to celebrate her first major weight loss? Prior to that, she had admitted to eating a pretty refined diet.

Redeeming quality: As consumers have become more savvy about health and nutrition, food manufactures have started enriching refined products with nutrients, though it hardly replaces what has been lost.

Remember: Breads, rice, and pasta all come in whole-grain versions, but just don't go by their darker color as that can be deceiving. Make sure the word "whole" appears on the package.

COFFEE

I know, I know, it's a toughie. As much as we all adore the daily grind, caffeine stimulates the adrenal glands to release the stress hormone cortisol to produce a short-term spike of alertness referred to as "flight or fight." The cortisol stimulates the liver to break down glycogen, raising your blood sugar level. Then the pancreas responds by releasing insulin to bring the blood sugar back down, making you more tired than before. For you diehard addicts who just can't get off the java, try organic freshly roasted coffee which tastes less bitter than regular coffee, and limit your intake to one or two cups max a day.

Major yuck factor: Cortisol has also been linked to belly fat.

Redeeming quality: Starbucks or Tim Hortons for the Canadians like me.

Visit: Your local health store and try the root of the chicory plant as a substitute. It delivers the electrolyte potassium in a readily absorbable liquid form that stimulates the rapid transmission of nerve impulses. You'll get the rush without the crash.

SODIUM

Sodium is the chief ingredient in table salt, but it shows up just about everywhere—not just in prepared foods like soup, but also in baking soda, seasonings, condiments, and, believe it or not, antacids, and even some prescription and over-the-counter drugs. Sodium is necessary to regulate muscle contraction, fluid balance, and nerve impulses in the human body, but the problem is that we eat three to 10 times the daily amount. This increases the chance of developing high blood pressure, which in turn can raise your risk of heart disease, kidney disease, and stroke. Even though salt has no calories, it's a chief cause of water retention—think of those 3 pounds that show up out of nowhere, overnight, when you hardly ate anything the night before! (It's been said you retain three times the weight in water of the sodium you ingest.) Many crash diets have foods with little or no salt content, but the weight loss that results is water loss. As soon as you eat foods containing salt, the weight comes back. And that's just evil.

Major yuck factor: Sodium nitrate is added to processed meats to fight botulism. Just imagine the harshness unleashed in the body.

Redeeming quality: Foods labeled "sodium free," "low sodium," or "reduced sodium."

Remember: Sodium is found naturally in most foods, and table salt is 40 percent sodium. Adding salt is overkill. Your best bet is to cook from scratch without it, and if you must, use unrefined sea salt with its large mineral content sparingly. Or find other ways of adding flavor (see Jennifer's Rock Star Spice Rack) and avoid processed foods.

ARTIFICIAL SWEETENERS

The fact that they were created to be used in a diabetic diet should make them okay, right? 'Fraid not. One of the most common ones, Aspartame (NutraSweet, Equal), is actually made of formaldehyde and has been linked to brain cancer in rats. Saccharin (Sweet 'n' Low) has also been linked to cancer and has been banned in Canada, although it is still used in food in the U.S. The conventional wisdom is that these should all be safe enough when used in moderation. The problem is that more and more of them are showing up or actually hidden in our foods. We really don't know how much of them we are ingesting. If you must, the best bet seems to be sucralose (Splenda) as it passes through the body unchanged and is therefore a noncaloric sweetener. Also stevia, derived from a South American shrub, is becoming popular among people who like its natural provenance. Although it is not allowed in food in the U.S., Canada, and the European Union as there are toxicity concerns, it is widely available in many health food stores. Its supporters say that it has been used in Japan for three decades without any side effects, while the naysayers point out that it is used in very few foodstuffs, and then just sparingly. Proceed with very small amounts and caution.

Major yuck factor: The word "artificial" says it all.

Redeeming quality: They have a fraction of the calories of sugar.

Remember: You are not a kid at a party: That sweet tooth does not necessarily have to be indulged.

HIGH-FRUCTOSE CORN SYRUP

I've saved the worst for last. High in calories and low in nutritional value, this is the sweetener and preservative used in fruit-flavored drinks, sodas, and in way more packaged goods than is healthy. This is very high on the evil meter as fructose is more easily converted into fat than other sugars, increasing its presence in the bloodstream. It has also been linked to diabetes and high cholesterol, so don't drink up. Also try to stay away from sugar and its derivatives like sucrose, maltose, dextrose, lactose, and fructose. Especially in its refined form, I consider sugar to be one of the most destructive legal drugs on the market, right up there with nicotine! Sugar has been linked to everything from migraines to mood disorders and, of course, weight gain. You do not need it—we get more than enough natural sugars in complex carbohydrates (see Principle 3).

Major yuck factor: The obscene childhood obesity epidemic has been linked directly to this substance.

Redeeming quality: Absolutely nothing.

Remember: Whole fruits and natural fruit juices give you all the sugar you need without the poisonous side effects.

PRINCIPLE 5: HOW LOW CAN YOU GO? EAT ACCORDING TO THE GLYCEMIC INDEX

The Glycemic Index (G.I.) is a system that was created to measure how much a particular carbohydrate affects your blood sugar level. The body breaks down carbohydrates into simple sugars, which it then uses for energy. The G.I. gives each food a number from one to 100 to determine the effect it may have on your body and is classified as high, medium, or low. Naturally, sugar is the standard measurement to which all foods are compared; it has a G.I. rating of 100 as it significantly raises your blood sugar level. Foods that rate high (with a G.I. above 70) are quickly absorbed into the bloodstream, causing your blood sugar levels to spike immediately, then quickly drop. So while you will feel immediately satiated and have an energy surge, you will crash and soon be hungry again. That hunger will take the form of sugar cravings. This is how the sugar addiction manifests itself. All leading nutritionists now agree that including foods with a medium or low G.I. rating in each meal is the best way to control and eliminate this cycle. Those foods will provide a continuing source of energy as the rise in your blood sugar level will be gradual. In other words, your hunger and cravings will be stabilized and there will be no more "I've gotta have it" drama!

THE GLYCEMIC INDEX RATING OF COMMON FOODS

High (more than 70)
Glucose 100
Baked potato 85
Bagel 72
Pretzels 83
Rice cakes 82
Doughnuts 75
Watermelon 72
White bread 70

Moderate (56 to 69)
Orange juice 57
Basmati Rice 58
Coucous 65
Popcorn 55
Pineapple 66
Mango 60
Figs 61

Low (less than 55)
Brown rice 55
Corn 55
Sweet potato 54
Banana 54
Apple juice 41
Apple 36
Skim milk 32
Green beans 30
Lentils 29
Garbonzo beans 28
Grapefruit 25
Broccoli 15
Strawberries 40
Cherries 22

GLYCEMIC INDEX CHART OF FOODS

Recommended Food Categories	Glycemic Index Average(GI)	Recommended Food Categories	Glycemic Index Average(GI)
Apples	Low	*Breads*	
Beans	Low	White Bread	High
Vegetables	Low	Pumpernickel Bread	Low
Dairy	Low	Rye Bread	High
Oatmeal and other oats	Low	Flaxseed	Low
Sweet Potato	Low to Moderate	Oat Bran	Low
Meats and Proteins	None	Pita Bread	Med
Legumes	Low	Wonder White Bread	High
Cereals very low in Sugar	Low to Moderate	Whole Wheat Tortillas	Med
		Sourdough	Low
Beverages			
Beer	Moderate	*Breakfast Breads*	
Coffee	No effect	All Bran	Low
Gatorade and other Sports Drinks	High	Bran Flakes	High
		Coco Pops	High
		Froot Loops	Med

Recommended Food Categories	Glycemic Index Average(GI)	Recommended Food Categories	Glycemic Index Average(GI)
Frosted Flakes	Med	Prunes	Low
Muesli	Low	Raisins	Med
Nutri-Grain	Med		
Instant Oatmeal	High	*Fresh Fruit*	
Steel Cut Oats	Low	Apples	Low
Puffed Rice	High	Apricots	Med
Raisin Bran	High	Avocados	VERY Low
Rice Krispies	High	Banana	Low
Shredded Wheat	High	Canteloupe	Med
Special K	Med	Cherries	Med
		Grapefruit	Low
Muffins and Cakes		Grapes	Low
Angel Food Cake	Med	Kiwi	Low
Banana Bread	Low	Mango	Low
Blueberry Muffin	Med	Orange	Low
Carrot Muffin	Med	Papaya	Med
Croissant, plain	Med	Peach	Low
Cupcake	High	Pear	Low
Pancakes from premade package	Med to High	Pineapple	Med
Waffles	High	Strawberries	Low
		Watermelon	High
Cereal Grains			
Buckwheat	Low	*Meat*	
Millet	High	Bacon	None
Quinoa	Low	Beef Lean	None
Bulgur	Low	Calamari	None
Polenta	Med	All Fish	None
		Chicken nuggets Breaded	Low
ALL DAIRY PRODUCTS	Low	Seafood	None
		Fish Sticks	None
Fruit Dried		Ham	None
Apples	Low	Lamb	None
Apricots	Low	Lobster	None
Cranberries, sweetened	Med	Turkey	None
Dates	Low to Med	Tuna	None
Figs	Med	Sushi	Low

Recommended Food Categories	Glycemic Index Average(GI)	Recommended Food Categories	Glycemic Index Average(GI)
Pastas		Life Savers	High
Fettuccine egg noodles cooked	Low	Corn Chips, Plain, Salted	Low
Gnocchi, cooked	Med	Dark Chocolate	Low
Instant noodles	Med		
Linguine	Low	*Spreads*	
Macaroni and Cheese	Med	Honey	Low
		Agave	Low
Rice		Jam (100% fruit)	Low
Basmati Rice	Med	Nutella, hazlenut spread	Med
Brown Rice	Med		
Instant Rice	High	*Vegetables*	
Jasmine Rice	High	Most vegetables have a low GI,	
Long Grain	Low	we will show you the others	
Wild Rice	Med	Beets, red, canned	Med
		Broad Beans (fava)	High
Candy		Carrots (cooked)	Low to Med
Jelly Beans	High	Parsnips	High
Licorice, soft	High	Potato	High
		Peas	Low

PRINCIPLE 6: LET GO: EAT LIKE THERE IS NO TOMORROW BECAUSE THERE ISN'T

Something has to give, so I recommend a little cheating. This is a day-long time-out, once a week, when you can eat anything you like. The irony is eventually you won't want to. In my experience, as people see Rock Star Fitness results and feel the effects of the eating principles, they are less inclined to tuck into that large oil-popped popcorn slathered in trans-fatty butter on a weekly basis! For instance, Linda Evangelista cheated once a year with a burger and fries. At some point, eating well will become a way of life and you will get used to that way of life and come to love it. When you do take a time-out, you will not want to waste it on junk. Instead, you'll opt for a great bottle of red wine or a fabulous gourmet meal. That's worth it. Or you'll save your

Fiber, which is also known as roughage, is a headline act in Rock Star eating. It is a plant carbohydrate and cannot be digested, but it keeps the digestive system functioning properly by speeding up the elimination of waste. There are two types of fiber. Insoluble fiber prevents constipation and therefore allows toxins to leave the body as quickly as possible. Soluble fiber also performs this function while also lowering the level of cholesterol in the bloodstream and slowing down the digestion and the sudden release of sugar in the bloodstream. Also, because fiber is low in calories and bulky, you are left feeling fuller longer, making fiber an excellent food for weight loss and maintenance.

Insoluble fibre sources: All bran, wholemeal flour and bread, brown rice, whole-grain cereals, vegetables, edible fruit skin, nuts and seeds

Soluble fiber sources: Fruits, vegetables, lentils, peas, beans, oats, barley, oatmeal, dried fruit, and soy meal

Eat up to 2 ounces of fiber a day. If this is an increase for you, drink more water to avoid constipation. Also start taking a multivitamin if you don't already do so as essential minerals such as zinc, calcium, and iron can be eliminated from the body along with the fiber before they are absorbed into the bloodstream.

cheating for a real occasion like on your birthday. You will enjoy getting older a lot more when you begin to be your best self, your body leading the way. By that time you will have realized that eating healthily tastes and looks better.

DECODING THE LABEL

Three important pieces of information can be found on the labels of most packaged foods to help you make better choices toward good health:

1. *The nutrition facts panel:* This states the serving size, the amount of calories, and the nutrients of food. It's important to remember that all of this information applies to one serving. If a serving is 1 cup and you eat 2 cups, you consume twice the calories and other nutrients given on the label.

2. *The ingredient list:* On packaged food this gives an overview of the "recipe," which is especially useful for people with allergies or food sensitivities Ingredients are listed in descending order by weight. For example, Kellogg's Raisin Bran cereal lists whole wheat as the first ingredient, which indicates it contains more whole wheat than anything else. Make sure that those first three or four ingredients are healthy choices. If sugar (or any of its variations) is second or third on the list, step away from the package!

3. *Nutrient content claims:* Nutrient content claims—such as "low-fat," "high-fiber," or "saturated fat-free"—are strictly defined by the government for a single serving and are a quick way to identify foods with a specific nutritional feature. Use this table as your guide to nutrient content claims:

YOUR CHEATING HEART

You're not alone. Here's how celebrities fall off the wagon.

Carrie Underwood: Pumpkin pie
Vanessa Hudgens: Chocolate
Jenny McCarthy: Cold Stone ice cream cake
Angie Harmon: Stuffing and gravy
Stacy Keibler: Ice cream
Regina King: Absolut Vodka pear martinis
Haylie Duff: Tortilla chips and salsa
Carmen Electra: Pizza and bakery goods, especially cupcakes and icing
Cameron Diaz: French fries

Notice how the temptations fall into the sweet, salty, or creamy categories. Now here are my favorite crave-busting, fit-friendly substitutes.

If you're craving something sweet:
Cottage cheese with diced fruits make a super-yummy snack. Choose low-fat cottage cheese and mix in pineapples, blueberries, strawberries, and apples with their good natural sugars. Add slivered almonds for extra protein and crunch.
Sliced apples with almond butter will also do the trick.

If you're craving something salty:
Hummus with pita is a great alternative to fattening, overprocessed dips. You can buy it from the store or create your own by blending chickpeas with a touch of olive oil and garlic. Then cut whole-wheat pitas into slivers and bake in the oven until crunchy. Oven-roasted pita chips taste great, fill you up with fiber—and all without sodium.

If you're craving something rich and creamy:
Add fruits and nuts to plain yogurt. When shopping for yogurt, look for the words "live culture" or "pro-biotic yogurt." (Another great option is Greek yogurt, which is always made from live cultures.) This assures that the yogurt has maintained the good bacteria that help to break down lactose (milk sugars) and keep the digestive track working well.

Also try low-fat or skim-milk cheeses such as Laughing Cow Baby Bell cheese or Kraft String Cheese. It's low in calories and high in calcium, but still has a comparatively high percentage of fat. One packet should be enough to quell the craving.

And speaking of savvy substitutes for weight loss, stop being nutty and go to seed instead. Nuts are quite calorically dense; for instance, only 15 cashews have a whopping 180 calories. And on top of that, it is very tough not to overeat these imminently munchable snacks. Consider switching to seeds because they are much higher in protein than most nuts. With protein being 4 calories a gram and fat being 9, you can see why you should.

NUTS

Almonds: 100 grams contain 16.9 grams protein, 4.2 milligrams iron, 250 milligrams calcium, 20 milligrams vitamin E, 3.1 milligrams zinc, and 0.92 milligrams vitamin B2.
Brazil nuts: 100 grams contain 12 grams protein, 61 grams fat, 2.8 milligrams iron, 180 milligrams calcium, and 4.2 milligrams zinc.
Cashews: 100 grams contain 17.2 grams protein, 60 micrograms vitamin A, 3.8 milligrams iron.

SEEDS

Sunflower seeds: 100 grams also contain 24 grams protein, 7.1 milligrams iron, and 120 milligrams calcium.
Pumpkin seeds: 100 grams contain 29 grams protein, 11.2 milligrams iron, and 1,144 milligrams phosphorous.
Sesame seeds: 100 grams contain 26.4 grams protein, 12.6 milligrams vitamin B3, 7.8 milligrams iron, 131 milligrams calcium, and 10.3 milligrams zinc.

Nutrient Content Claim	Definition (per serving)
Calorie-free	Less than 5 calories
Low-calorie	40 calories or less
Reduced or fewer calories	At least 25 percent fewer calories*
Light or lite	Calories reduced by at least one-third (if food is less than 50 percent calories from fat)
Sugar	
Sugar-free	Less than 0.5 gram sugars
Reduced sugar or less sugar	At least 25 percent less sugars*
No added sugar	No sugars added during processing or packing, including ingredients that contain sugars, such as juice or dried fruit
Fat	
Fat-free	Less than 0.5 gram fat
Low-fat	3 grams or less of fat
Reduced or less fat	At least 25 percent less fat*
Light or lite	Fat reduced 50 percent or more (if food is 50 percent or more calories from fat)
Saturated Fat	
Saturated fat-free	Less than 0.5 gram saturated fat and less than 0.5 gram trans fat
Low saturated fat	1 gram or less saturated fat and no more than 15 percent of calories from saturated fat
Reduced or less saturated fat	At least 25 percent less saturated fat
Cholesterol	
Cholesterol-free	Less than 2 milligrams cholesterol and 2 grams or less of saturated fat

Nutrient Content Claim	Definition (per serving)
Low cholesterol	20 milligrams or less per reference amount (and per 50 grams of food if the reference amount is small) 2 grams or less saturated fat per reference amount
Reduced or less cholesterol	At least 25 percent less cholesterols and 2 grams or less saturated fat
Sodium	
Sodium-free	Less than 5 milligrams sodium
Very low sodium	35 milligrams or less sodium
Low sodium	140 milligrams or less sodium
Reduced or less sodium	At least 25 percent less sodium
Light in sodium	50 percent less*
Fiber	
High-fiber	5 grams or more
Good source of fiber	2.5–4.9 grams more or added fiber at least 2.5 grams more* Other claims: high, rich in, excellent source of 20 percent or more of % Daily Value* Good source, contains, provides 10–19 percent of % Daily Value* More, enriched, fortified, added 10 percent or more of % Daily Value*
Lean**	Less than 10 grams fat, 4.5 grams or less saturated fat, and 95 milligrams cholesterol
Extra lean**	Less than 5 grams fat, 2 grams saturated fat, and 95 milligrams cholesterol as compared with a standard serving size of the traditional food
** on meat, poultry, seafood, and game meats ***source: Kelloggs	

DEVIL INSIDE

And remember:

1. Many foods that appear to come in a single-sized serving might contain as many as three times that amount. Before you open that package, check the label's serving size, so you are aware of what the limits are.

2. Pay particular attention to the calories you eat, and not just the fat content, as many foods that are labeled "light" or "low-fat" may still be high in calories, or be labeled "low-carb" but be high in fat.

3. Total fat means the total amount of fat per serving. It generally includes both the amount of saturated fat and trans fats. Look for foods with less than a gram of saturated fat per serving (1 gram of fat = 9 calories).

4. Total carbohydrates means the combined amount of sugar, complex carbohydrates, and fiber in a serving (1 gram of carbs = 4 calories).

5. Protein is the total amount of protein found in a food, measured in grams (1 gram of protein = 4 calories).

6. The percentage of your daily vitamin and mineral requirements is listed, based on a 2,000 calorie-a-day diet.

7. You should limit your sodium intake to no more than 2.3 grams (2,300 milligrams) per day. Compare the amount listed to the serving size and remember this is also based on a 2,000 calorie-a-day diet.

JENNIFER'S ROCK STAR SUPERFOODS

What makes a Rock Star a Superstar? They have it all and they deliver more; they simply take it to the next level. This describes my Rock Star superfoods. Within each is a medley of necessities that hit every nutritional note. I have chosen them specifically because they are packed with vitamins and minerals that are key to health, but are sadly lacking in many North American diets. They also provide power fuel through protein and complex carbs, and most importantly—and what truly makes them super—is their antioxidant content. Try very, very, very hard to include these foods in your diet as the beauty, health, and fitness benefits to you will be enormous.

AMARANTH

Why: This nutty-tasting grain gives you nearly double the protein and three times as much fiber as brown rice for about the same number of calories.

Super Power: One of the only nonmeat sources of all nine amino acids—the building blocks of protein—that the body uses to create muscle. It's also high in nutrients like iron, zinc, and calcium.

Fab Fact: The Ancient Aztecs believed that eating amaranth could actually give them superpowers!

APPLE

Why: One of my all-time favorite snacks, they are very low cal and their infinite variety—they go from tart to sweet—will satisfy every craving.

Super Power: A source of both soluble and insoluble fiber, apples will guard against arteriosclerosis and heart disease, while keeping your system regular and acting as a natural mouth freshener. Eat with the skin—that's where all the vitamin C is stored!

Fab Fact: Eating an apple has been proven to extend workout energy by 10 minutes.

ASPARAGUS

Why: This is a miracle vegetable that is low in calories, fat, sodium, and high in fiber and antioxidants.

Super Power: A rich source of folic acid that fights against cancer and heart disease. A mild diuretic, asparagus is also a natural detoxifier, while at the same time it promotes healthy bacteria in the stomach, so it fights bloating.

Fab Fact: It's a known libido lifter as folates are linked to the creation of histamines, which are essential to orgasm.

YOU WANT THIS

Vitamins and minerals are micronutrients that work with your body to help extract energy from the foods you eat, and also ensure that your body performs at an optimum level. Vitamins and minerals perform many tasks in your body, including digestion, transporting nutrients, regulating muscle contraction, maintaining water balance, and aiding in absorption.

WHAT YOU NEED

Antioxidants, or vitamins A, C, E, and beta-carotene, are found in orange, red, yellow, and green fruits and vegetables. They protect the body from free radical damage. Free radicals occur, causing cellular breakdown, through normal biological functions and the aging process and can be exacerbated by environmental factors such as stress, sun damage, and alcohol, as well as processed and sugary foods. Free radical damage is at the root of cancer and the biggest culprit of premature aging, which starts from the inside out. So not only will antioxidants keep you healthy internally, they are also major beauty boosters that keep the skin looking younger longer, and hair and nails healthy.

AVOCADO

Why: Avocado is a fruit rich in monounsaturated fat—the good kind.

Super Power: Loaded with a variety of disease-fighting antioxidants—vitamins A, B, C, and E, it also boasts vitamin K, which, among other things, builds bone and helps fight off osteoporosis so it is key for women; potassium, which is necessary for nerve function, muscle control, and high blood pressure; as well as iron.

Fab Fact: Pairing avocados with other fruits and vegetables helps the body better absorb their antioxidants.

CHERRIES

Why: Cherries are tasty with natural sugars that pack a powerful antioxidant punch.

Super Power: They fight inflammation as they boast compounds similar to Aspirin and ibuprofen. They are rich with potassium; calcium, which fights osteoporosis; magnesium, which fights excessive belly fat, insulin resistance, and elevated blood pressure; and iron, which oxygenates the blood and muscles, and supports collagen, which keeps the skin elastic and the immune system healthy. And if that's not enough, cherries are great intestinal sweepers!

Fab Fact: Cherries raise the level of melatonin in the body, which improves the body's circadian rhythms and therefore sleep patterns.

GARLIC

Why: Garlic is potent not just because of its infamous scent, but also for its legendary health benefits.

Super Power: It boosts your body's own supply of hydrogen sulfide, which acts as an antioxidant to increase blood flow. Garlic also staves off various cancers and lowers cholesterol levels, and fights off colds and flu. Crush the garlic at room temperature and allow it to sit for about 15 minutes before cooking. This gives the enzyme reaction that triggers garlic's healthy time for maximum impact.

Fab Fact: The ancient Greeks would feed garlic to their athletes before they competed in the Olympic Games.

GRAPEFRUIT

Why: Research has shown that eating half a grapefruit before a meal will aid weight loss.

Super Power: All grapefruits are packed with cancer-fighting compounds, but the red grapefruit has been shown to help lower triglycerides, the blood fats that can lead to heart disease.

Fab Fact: Half a grapefruit has only 39 calories!

GREEN VEGETABLES

Why: Lettuce and spinach, broccoli and cabbage, as well as alfalfa sprouts are full of antioxidants.

Super Power: Rapini, also known as broccoli rabe, is pleasingly bitter, and contains a quarter of the calories of the better-known broccoli (at only 9 calories per cup!) and twice the amount of vitamin A. It is also a good source of folate, vitamin K, and beta-carotene, and has a protective effect against stomach, lung, and breast cancers. Swiss chard, like a crunchy spinach, boasts only 7 calories per cup and contains vision-protecting lutein, vitamin A, and beta-carotene, but Swiss chard has twice the amount of vitamin K as spinach. Just 1 cup provides more than three times the daily dose of the nutrient.

Fab Fact: They also detoxify your body while boosting your immune system.

IT'S SO EASY BEING GREEN

I believe that a salad should form the core of every meal, especially at night. They fill you up, are extremely low cal (just make sure your dressing is too so you don't defeat the purpose), and they will help keep you regular. The biggest problem with salad is getting stuck in a leafy rut, so here is the ultimate "green" mix-it-up ingredient list:

What It's Called	Calorie Count Per Cup	What It Looks Like and How It Tastes	How to Choose It	How to Prepare it
Belgian endive	9	4–6 inch long tapered bundles; leaves are creamy white with yellow tips; is slightly bitter, but its crunchy bite makes it addictive.	Avoid browning edges as they are extra bitter; store wrapped in a paper towel inside fridge to extend shelf life.	Cut the endive in half lengthwise or use whole leaves as an edible scoop; is great with pears and nuts in an Asian salad.
Bibb, Boston or butterhead lettuce	8	Small, round, and loosely formed heads and buttery soft leaves; prized for its sweet, subtle taste.	Check the leaves are firmly attached; handle gently; lasts a week in the fridge.	Goes great with all other greens; dress it with vinaigrette or olive oil and lemon juice.
Bok choy	10	Is in the cabbage family; wide white stocks and full green leaves; crunchy, mild, and juicy.	Refrigerate in a perforated plastic bag for long life; look for large-leaf variety.	Is great in coleslaws and stir-fries; is great with seared seafood or chicken.
Cabbage (red, green and curly)	22	Is one of the world's healthiest plants that fights cancer; sweet and crisp flavor; supplies 100 percent recommended daily allowance of vitamin C!	Look for heads that are heavy and solid with only a few loose leaves; avoid cracks or brown spots.	Is great shredded into coleslaw or made into soups or cabbage rolls.
Chicory/curly endive	21	Very curly green leaves and a pale heart; it has 4 grams of fiber per cup (twice the amount in other greens).	Best to buy small chicories as they get bitter as they grow old; store in airtight container.	Has a very strong flavor so it's best mixed with other greens; lovely served with garlic.

What It's Called	Calorie Count Per Cup	What It Looks Like and How It Tastes	How to Choose It	How to Prepare it
Chinese cabbage	13	Dark green, long and narrow with leaf tips fanning out that are very wrinkled; sweet and tender flavor.	Look for crisp leaves with no sign of browning; lasts up to two weeks!	Is excellent cooked in soups and stir-fries; is tasty eaten raw in coleslaws and salads; pair with spicy foods.
Collard greens	25	It looks like a cross between a kale and cabbage with long, flat green leaves; mild flavor that is high in vitamin C.	Look for small, firm, and bright green collards; avoid yellow or leaves with holes.	Is very popular in the southern parts of the United States; stack leaves in a pile and cut fine; steam lightly.
Green and red leaf lettuce	5	It does not have a head; it has loose, delicate leaves that are very flavorful.	Soak in cold water to clean and store in paper towels inside plastic to preserve up to a week.	Is delicious with grapefruit, onion, and mustard vinaigrette; add dressing right before to prevent wilting.
Iceberg lettuce	7	The lowest in nutrition of all the greens; has bland taste.	Look for the darkest leaves possible to boost nutrition; choose only when there is nothing else available.	It is nice if you want something very mild to cut spice, like in tacos.
Kale (available in dino, purple, and flowering)	11	Is in the cabbage family; has a crisp texture and mild flavor; large, ruffled-edged green leaves.	Select firm, crisp leaves and refrigerate for up to a week.	Pairs well with strong flavors like garlic, and ginger; is best steamed or used in a stir-fry.
Radicchio (pronounced Rad-EEK-ee-o)	12	A red chicory that has a bittersweet, satin finish; is a favorite of gourmet chefs.	Turn over to look at the core; avoid if there are signs of browning; lasts up to one week in the fridge.	Remove the core with a sharp knife and separate the leaves; pairs with beans, nuts, olives, and fish.

What It's Called	Calorie Count Per Cup	What It Looks Like and How It Tastes	How to Choose It	How to Prepare it
Romaine lettuce	4	Has taken over iceberg as everyone's go-to green; is sweet with a great crunch.	Look for leaves with no brown spots; it will last longer if you wash before storage; use a paper towel in a tight plastic bag.	Is wonderful as a base for any salad; made famous by Caesar salad, but works well with Mandarin oranges and slivered almonds.
Spinach	40	Sweet and loaded with iron, calcium, and vitamins A, B, and C	Choose crisp, dark leaves; avoiding any yellowing; use in three days; if short on time, go for baby spinach that is pre-washed.	Substitute for lettuce in salads to boost nutrition; pairs well with berries and mushrooms.
Watercress	4	A delicate green with a peppery bite; is a member of the mustard family with fragile stems and small green leaves.	Look for fresh leaves with deep-green color; avoid yellowing or wilted leaves; lasts only a day, so eat up.	Cut off tips of stems and rinse well; the peppery taste is great for a topping to salads or soups.

HEMP SEEDS

Why: Contains a highly digestible form of whole protein.

Super Power: They are an excellent source of the rare gamma-linoleic acid (GLA), which is important for protecting us from degenerative conditions like arthritis. GLA also lowers cholesterol and balances hormonal activity. And to top things off nicely, as hemp seeds do for yogurts and salads, hemp seeds are cholesterol-free!

Fab Fact: A scoop contains half of your daily requirement of EFAs.

KIWIS

Why: Kiwis are fat-, sodium-, and cholesterol-free. Research shows that among 27 different fruits, the little kiwi is the most nutritionally dense per calorie. That is, they have the highest concentration of vitamins and minerals, with more vitamin C than oranges and grapefruits, and more potassium than bananas.

Super Power: Next to dark, leafy greens, kiwis are one of the top sources of lutein, an antioxidant that is important for vision and heart health. In another study it was concluded that healthy adults who ate two kiwi fruits a day for a month lowered their triglycerides by 15 percent. Kiwi also boasts an impressive amount of fiber for its size.

Fab Fact: Because of the enzyme actinidin, kiwi is a natural meat tenderizer.

LEMON AND LIMES

Why: Rich in vitamin C, they are natural detoxifiers for the blood and liver.

Super Power: Full of potent plant chemicals, they lower the risk of arthritis, stroke, cancer, and heart disease while shoring up the immune system. They are also helpful in maintaining the body's acidic/alkaline balance.

Fab Fact: The tartness of lemons and limes can trick the taste buds into not wanting as much salt.

OATS

Why: One of nature's most nutritious cereals, it provides loads of energy with nerve-fortifying ingredients.

Super Power: With their high-fiber content, oats are an excellent food in lowering cholesterol and reducing the risk of heart disease. They are also rich in complex carbohydrates that are linked to reducing cancer and controlling diabetes. With some protein, some good fats, B-vitamins (which are important for beauty and the breakdown of nutrients), and vitamin E, oats are also mineral rich.

Fab Fact: They are also considered a cleansing grain that detoxifies the intestines and the blood.

FINDING BALANCE

You may wonder why something as acidic as lemons and limes will help keep the body balanced with alkalinity, but a food's acid or alkaline-forming tendency does not correlate with the food's pH balance itself but to its end products after digestion. So in this case the body figuratively takes lemons and makes lemonade. The body's acidic/alkaline or PH balance is very important to health and fitness as overacidity of the tissues has been linked to a host of conditions, including weight gain, increased free radical production, premature aging, low energy, osteoporosis, joint pain, slow digestion and elimination, as well as cardiovascular disease. Unfortunately, the average North American diet is rife with acid-forming foods and products that tend to be the usual suspects. They have to be neutralized with foods and products that cause alkalinity for proper balance. Naturopaths suggest that the diet should consist of at least 60 percent alkaline-forming foods and, at most, 40 percent acid-forming foods.

Acid-Forming Foods: Meat, eggs, dairy, refined flour, refined sugar, coffee, soft drinks, and artificial sweeteners.

Alkaline-Forming Foods: Beans, legumes, green leafy vegetables, apples, pears, bananas, herb teas, complex carbs like sweet potatoes and wild rice, nuts, flaxseed oil, and olive oil.

PINEAPPLE

Why: This tropical fruit is rich in the enzyme group bromelian, which breaks down protein and aids digestion in the intestinal tract.

Super Power: A source of dietary fiber, pineapple also has vitamins B1 and B6 for energy production, immune support, and copper, which supports energy metabolism.

Fab Fact: Stocks the mineral manganese, which has been shown to reduce osteoporosis.

PUMPKIN

Why: The pumpkin is a fiber-rich vegetable that is too good to be saved just for Thanksgiving.

Super Power: It is a great source of vitamins K, and E, and lots of minerals, including magnesium, potassium, and iron. Pumpkin is also loaded with vitamins A, C, and other powerful antioxidants.

Fab Fact: It is so low cal and low fat that pumpkin is even allowed during the draconian Atkins induction phase.

QUINOA

Why: Quinoa is a health-giving seed of a leafy plant (it's related to beets, spinach, and Swiss chard).

Super Power: It is rich in protein (considered to be complete due to the presence of all eight essential amino acids), calcium, and a good source of vitamins E and B. It is versatile as a breakfast cereal or as a grain-like ingredient in soups and stews.

Fab Fact: In South America, quinoa is used as a topical treatment for burns and cuts.

SARDINES

Why: Sardines are a fantastic source of omega-3s.

Super Power: Sardines are also loaded with protein, which helps stabilize blood sugar, makes you feel full, and helps stimulate metabolism.

Fab Fact: They are so small and low on the food chain with a low life expectancy that their toxicity level is extremely low, especially when compared to farm tuna.

WALNUTS

Why: Although they contain more fat per 1 ounce serving than almonds (18 grams versus 14), the majority of fat is from omega-3 fatty acids.

Super Power: Walnuts are also high in sterols, which are plant compounds that inhibit the absorption of cholesterol. Research shows that eating walnuts regularly can cause LDL (bad cholesterol) levels to drop by as much as 16 percent.

Fab Fact: Another study found that people who ate approximately 10 walnuts with a meal high in artery-clogging saturated fat experienced less harmful inflammation in their blood vessels than those who didn't have the nuts.

WHEAT GERM

Why: When eaten fresh and raw, it's the most nutritious portion of the wheat kernel (the area from which the seed germinates before it sprouts), and is a low-cal alternative to granola.

Super Power: It's rich in protein, vitamin B-complex, vitamin E enzymes, and minerals. It also contains octacosanol, which lowers cholesterol, aids energy storage in muscles, balances metabolism, enhances endurance, and aids in stress, among other things.

Fab Fact: Due to milling, wheat germ has a very reduced level of the gluten protein, which causes wheat allergies.

WHEAT GRASS

Why: In the family of cereal grasses that includes barley grass and alfalfa, it boasts the most potent nutritious and healing properties.

Super Power: Considered the ultimate supplement, it is fat- and cholesterol-free and protein-packed. It contains vitamins A, B-17,C, E, and K.

It also contains minerals including calcium, iron, and zinc, which is necessary for healthy skin, healing, and enzyme functions.

Fab Fact: Wheat grass is 70 percent chlorophyll, the pigment that captures light energy in plants and is almost chemically identical to hemoglobin, which carries oxygen from the lungs to the body's tissues. This makes wheat grass a body cleanser, anti-inflammatory, and, what many believe, a fierce cancer fighter.

WILD SALMON

Why: Salmon is one of the best sources of omega-3s, but ensuring that it is wild, not farmed, will allow you to enjoy it while lowering the risk of ingesting toxic chemicals. Two servings a week of fatty fish like salmon are now recommended as part of a balanced diet.

Super Power: Reduces the risk of heart disease and stroke, but also Alzheimer's disease and depression. In addition to being an excellent source of omega-3s, salmon also has lots of selenium, protein, niacin, and vitamin B12, and is a good source of phosphorous, magnesium, and vitamin B6.

Fab Fact: Research shows that a larger number of omega-3s are absorbed through cooked salmon than cod liver oil supplement, even when more of the supplement is taken.

JENNIFER'S ROCK STAR SPICE RACK

In addition to making food tastier, herbs and spices are an abundant source of antioxidants and other health benefits. Adding a moderate amount of herbs and spices can go a long way to boosting the health value of a meal as they are low-cal, nutrient-packed substitutes for salt and artificial flavorings. But for real Rock Stars results, make sure you use them fresh: Fresh herbs and spices contain higher antioxidant levels compared to their processed counterparts. For example, the

---

TAKE ME HOME
And while you're at it, add these high-nutrient, low-cal items to your shopping cart:

Almonds
Balsamic vinegar
Black pepper
Brown rice
Extra-virgin olive oil
Low-sodium chicken broth
Low-sodium vegetable broth
Onions
Papaya
Rice vinegar
Snap peas
Sweet potatoes
Yams

antioxidant activity of fresh garlic is 1.5 times higher than dry garlic powder. Spice up your life with a few of my favorites.

Basil: With a whopping percentage of vitamin K, basil is more than just the secret weapon in pesto. It also gives DNA protection, has anti-inflammatory and antibacterial benefits, and promotes cardiovascular health.

Cinnamon: This anti-inflammatory supports digestive function, stimulates circulation, and stabilizes blood sugar while reducing cholesterol levels. It also constricts and tones tissues, relieves congestion, pain, and stiffness in muscles and joints as well as menstrual discomfort. It also helps prevent urinary tract infections, tooth decay, and gum disease.

Cloves: Their aromatic flavor masks a host of healing benefits, including anti-inflammatory and antioxidant properties, relief from respiratory ailments, intestinal parasites, and muscle pain, while all the while encouraging mental focus.

Dill: With the ability to freshen the breath when chewed, dill is good for a lot more than just pickles. It also fights liver problems, intestinal gas, infection, bronchitis, colds and fever, and the loss of appetite.

Ginger: Its sharp, refreshing flavor adds kick while warming up the system, protecting against bacteria, soothing nausea, eliminating intestinal gas, and relieving dizziness.

Nutmeg: Who would have guessed that this festive herb has so many healing properties? It helps lower blood pressure and cholesterol, improves concentration and circulation, and calms insomnia, anxiety, muscle spasms, indigestion, and diarrhea.

Oregano: The grand master of herbs, oregano has three to 20 times higher antioxidant activity than other herbs. It has 42 times more antioxidant activity than apples, 30 times more than potatoes, 12 times more than oranges, and four times more than blueberries.

Peppermint: The therapeutic effects of peppermint have been known for eons. It inhibits the growth of bacteria, soothes the digestive tract, and relieves symptoms of allergies and asthma.

Rosemary: Contains an ingredient that fights off free radical damage to the brain, which puts up defenses to not just an aging brain but to Alzheimer's and strokes. It also soothes the nervous system and staves off sickness.

Tarragon: A mild diuretic with anesthetic qualities, it stimulates appetite, relieves intestinal gas, and even helps with rheumatism.

Thyme: A mineral-rich source of nutrients, thyme is known to relieve respiratory problems, including coughs, bronchitis, and chest congestion.

THE TOP FIVE:
Kitchen Tools for Tip-Top Shape

Cast-iron frying pan: This good old-fashioned tool is designed to be used with a little bit of oil so it saves you from extra fat! To really cut back, use an aerosol pump to diffuse oil into the frying pan.

Non-stick frying pan: This is one way to really cut oil out of the equation.

Measuring cups: This is the only way to get serious about portion control until you get used to the correct ones and can go by eye and instinct.

Blender: Instead of making do with junky sugary juices and sodium-laden soups, you can whip up healthy smoothies or blend homemade vegetable soups on your own.

Small plates: Studies have shown you'll eat less if you eat on a smaller plate! It turns out that you really do eat with your eyes first. A smaller plate will look more full, tricking your brain into thinking you're eating more than you are.

Sunday: Pick a day when you are not that busy, which is Sunday for most people, and prepare your meals and snacks for the week in advance. Then prepackage and freeze all these daily options so that you can grab and go when time is tight. This way you can not use the "too busy to cook" excuse for grabbing that greasy cafeteria lunch. You might want to also think about investing in environmentally friendly and reusable lunch containers to reduce unnecessary waste and pollution.

THE CHICKEN AND THE EGG

Omega-3 eggs are produced by altering the diet of the laying chickens. Their special diet consists of alfalfa, corn, and soybeans with up to 20 percent of it consisting of flaxseeds. Consider flaxseeds the secret weapon in making these omega-3 eggs healthier. Protein packed—there are 25 grams of protein in every 100 grams of flaxseeds, not to mention omega-3 essential fatty acids—they are also an internal cleanser of toxic metabolic waste and are thought to be extra-beneficial against breast cancer. Although the total fat and cholesterol level of an omega-3 egg remains the same as a "normal" egg, it's the type of fat that makes the difference. As you know, omega-3 essential fatty acids are the healthiest possible fats, and an omega-3 egg contains approximately 320 milligrams of omega-3 fats while a regular egg contains approximately 63 milligrams. The bottom line? Either way lay off the yolks most of the time.

JENNIFER'S ROCK STAR SNACK LIST

When I've got the munchies, these are my go-to options:

- 20 raw almonds
- 15 walnuts
- Sugar free Fudgsicles (not "no sugar added")
- Sugar free Jell-O
- Mozzarella string cheese
- Hummus, but make sure you find a low fat brand with a high-protein count. I like Wendy & Barb's, which is made with lemon juice so it's only 30 calories per 2 tbsps or just make it yourself with the recipe I provided (see menu)
- Edamame
- Celery with nut butter, like natural peanut or almond butter , for a protein and an essential fatty acid kick
- Air-popped popcorn with a teaspoon of Parmesan cheese for its fill-me-up volume
- An apple, which is simply the best use ever of 80 calories.

CHAPTER 4

ROCK YOUR BODY

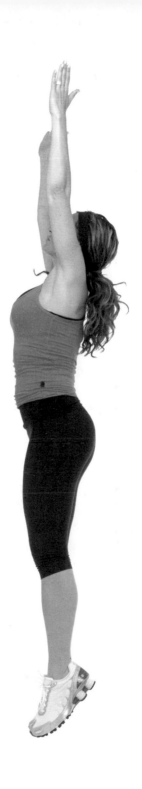

AND JUST AS SOPHIA LOREN FAMOUSLY quipped that she owed her sex siren curves to pasta, Madonna owes her Rock Star fabulousness to her hyper-disciplined routine of exercise. Back in the 1980s she transformed herself from a cuddly pop tart to a sleek, muscled power star, and she has never looked back. Her workout routines became as legendary as her reinventions and just like her, changed with the times. From 10-mile bike rides, to long jogs, to pumping iron, to hard-core yoga—and her perennial, dance—she did it all, and boy, does it ever show. At age 48, she successfully sported a leggings-and-leotard ensemble in her *Hung up* video and performed moves that most 25-year-olds would have a hard time pulling off. And it wasn't just the magic of digital imaging; she did it on live television as well. Now you might not want to have Madonna's Popcyc biceps, but there is no better example than Madonna of the benefits of a consistent commitment to exercise. Getting better with age and feeling and looking great along the way are pretty compelling incentives. It is the Rock Star way and you and I will walk it together. I have created an effective three-part program that will take you from so so to superfit and keep you there.

You will experience Ultimate Cardio and learn hot-body Power Moves. Then we'll put it all together in my Rock Star Boot Camp, which is a 14-day workout plan that will form the basis for what I know will be your ongoing fitness habit. Now we know what sort of habits folks in Hollywood can get up to, but this is the one every Rock Star should have.

GET INTO THE GROOVE

I have designed your Rock Star Program along two of the most effective and efficient training techniques: Interval Training for cardio and Circuit Training for resistance or muscle-building training.

Interval Training

Interval training alternates bursts of intense activity with intervals of lighter activity. It allows you to improve your aerobic capacity so you can exercise longer and harder. The higher-intensity intervals will cause you to burn more calories in the end. And it keeps you focused because you are constantly changing things up.

Circuit Training

An exercise circuit is a group of exercises designed to be completed one after the other in quick succession. Once you perform all the exercises, the circuit is complete. Then you start over again with the first exercise. I have designed your circuit to combine aerobic power bursts with muscle-building power moves so you can get the absolute most out of it.

BODY BASICS

Earlier I introduced you to the concept of different body types and asked you to identify yours to help you realize that we are meant to be different. And just like one body doesn't fit all, neither does an exercise regime. So it is important that you tweak Ultimate Cardio, Power Moves, and the 14-Day Rock Star Boot Camp to your particular fitness needs. Here's how.

Ectomorphs

Body Basics: Ectomorphs like Giselle are long and lean, have small bones, and a small percentage of fat and muscle. You don't gain weight easily, but when you do, it's not usually noticeable at first. You probably want to add lean muscle mass and curves.

Fit Tips Focus: Since ectomorphs have trouble gaining muscle, weight training is very important. And it is impossible for you to bulk up—you will look toned—so I would recommend using the heaviest weight you can comfortably handle for 6–10 reps. Do it, but go easy on the cardio. You never want to lose too much weight. Ectomorphs also typically have bad posture—all that slouching when you were the tallest girl in your class—so it's a good idea to include exercises that challenge the back muscles and shoulders. This will also give the illusion of more curves; a developed upper body makes the waist look smaller. By the way, yoga and Pilates are also great for posture. And remember, Ectos tend to have weaker bones, so gentle exercise is best.

Endomorphs

Body Basics: Endomorphs like Queen Latifah are round and soft—you often have more body fat than other types—and are larger in the face and hips. Endomorphs don't have trouble gaining muscle, but they do have a lot of trouble losing fat—it's in their genes. You probably want to burn fat.

Fit Tips Focus: Endomorphs should focus on high amounts of cardio exercise in order to burn the fat their bodies so easily store. Walk on an incline for a longer duration. If you are heavier, it will also be easier on the joints than running. When weight training, do higher reps with lighter weights instead of using heavier weights with lower repetitions. This will help you get toned rather than bulky, which is easy for you to do.

Mesomorphs

Body Basics: Mesomorphs, like Jessica Simpson and yours truly, have an athletic build. We have a high muscle mass, and have no trouble building more, and we also have strong bones. We are larger in the chest, but are typically lean all over. When we do gain weight, we do it in our midsection. We want to avoid bulking up.

Fit Tip Focus: Intense cardio workouts like sprints are effective. Try kickboxing as its intense cardio works the abs and obliques, which helps lean out the waist. Both cardio and strength training are equally important, but as Mesos also bulk up easily, do higher reps with lower weights

And, last but not least, as I mentioned way back in Chapter 2 when I introduced you to these categories, they are not necessarily strict pigeonholes. Some of you may have a blended body type, so use these tips as a guide and, if you must, blend them to make them work better for you. Now let's get moving.

MUSIC IS THE ANSWER

As I wrote in the introductory chapter to this book, one of my inspirations in developing my concept of Rock Star Fitness was the confidence and great sense of self that Rock Stars exude. And every one of them will tell you that it comes from the music, and how it makes them feel. From my own experience in working out and training others, I know how important music is to the experience and success of the session—the high and energy that can only come from the right playlist. This is especially necessary for you Rock Stars in the making. "Studies have shown that listening to music during exercise can improve results, both in terms of being a motivator (people exercise longer and more vigorously to music) and as a distraction from negatives like fatigue," says *The*

GET IN GEAR

Choose comfortable clothes because that is always the best choice for the best workout. I do believe that wearing something reasonably body conscious with supportive stretch fabrics gives a psychological lift. You should love and appreciate your body and see how it's working as you make it stronger.

But don't work out without the following:

- Garments made out of moisture-wicking microfiber fabric, which is also durable, lightweight, and chafe-free.
- A sports bra. They are designed to be ultra-supportive, but I like to buy them a little smaller so that it really holds me in.
- Professionally fitted running shoes. Runner stores offer this service and you should take them up on it. It is important that your instep and ankles are properly supported to avoid injury. Get new running shoes at least once a year as the support in them diminishes with wear and tear.

New York Times in "They're Playing My Song: Time to Work Out," their story on the issue.

Based on the research of Dr. Costas Karageorghis, an associate professor of sport psychology who rates music according to its "motivational qualities for various physical activities," *The Times* reported that the key factors for songs for working out are:

1. *The tempo:* It should be between 120 and 140 beats per minute (BPM), which coincides with the range of most commercial dance and rock music. "It also roughly corresponds to the average person's heart rate during a routine workout—say, 20 minutes on an elliptical trainer."

   In terms of BPMs for different activities, *The NY Times* compiled the list below based on Power Music compilations:

   - For a stroll walker going at a pace of around 3 miles an hour: 115–118 BPM.
   - For a power walker going 4.5 miles per hour: 137–139 BPM.
   - For a runner: 147–160 BPM.

2. *A consistent rhythm:* This aids coordination, the ability to synchronize your movements, and provides a timing cue, which "helps you to move more efficiently, which, in turn, can help you with endurance," not to mention enjoyment.

3. *Being loud and aggressive:* Especially when strength training or pumping iron, heavy metal or hip-hop "keeps you elevated, especially in between sets." In other words, the best music gives you a feeling that pushes you to keep going for it through pain and fatigue. According to Dr. Karageorghis, many opt for "Gonna Fly Now," the theme from Rocky, as it

"evokes a state of optimism and excitement in the listener," which for me and for you is really the bottom line: The music will move you, both figuratively and literally.

PUMP IT UP

When it's comes to really pumped up cardio it's all about more beats per minute, so when a song deserves an encore, go for the remix version. Dance remixes always have a faster, more intense tempo, much more beats per minutes than the original songs, which are quite fast to begin with. The remix is always great to help your really pump up your cardio!

PART 1: ULTIMATE CARDIO

JENNIFER'S WARM-YOU-UP/COOL-YOU-DOWN SONG PLAYLIST

"Tom's Diner," Suzanne Vega
"I'm Real," Jennifer Lopez
"What about Your Friends," TLC
"Read My Mind," The Killers
"When We Were Young," The Killers
"Beverly Hills," Weezer
"Sunday Shining," Finley Quaye
"Rich Girl," Gwen Stephani
"Umbrella," Rhianna
"Loungin'," LL Cool J
"Good life," Kayne West
"Because of you," Ne-Yo

The real deal about the ever so popular "FAT BURNING ZONE."

By now, you probably know that cardio is a key component in helping lose weight. Many people are told to stay within their "fat burning zone" but do you really burn more fat when you work in a

	Low Intensity - 60-65% MHR	High Intensity - 80-85% MHR
Total Calories expended per min.	4.86	6.86
Fat Calories expended per min.	2.43	2.7
Total Calories expended in 30 min.	146	206
Total Fat calories expended in 30 min.	73	82
Percentage of fat calories burned	50%	39.85%

From *The 24/5 Complete Personal Training Manual*, 24 Hour Fitness, 2000

JENNIFER"S ULTIMATE CARDIO PUMP-YOU-UP SONG PLAYLIST

"Maneater," Nelly Furtado (remix)
"Glamorous," Fergie
"Best of You," Foo Fighters
"Pretender," Foo Fighters
"I Don't Wanna be In love," Good Charlotte
"Viva la Vida," Coldplay
"Hot," Avril Lavigne
"Shake It," Metro Station
"Stand Back, "Stevie Nicks
"Thriller," Michael Jackson
"Wanna Be Starting Something," Michael Jackson
"Gimme More," Britney Spears
"Crazy," Britney Spears
"Everlong," Foo Fighters
"Indestructible," Mathew Good Band
"Write Sins Not Tragedies," Panic at the Disco
"When I Come around," Green Day
"Relax, Take It Easy," Mika
"It's my Life," Bon Jovi
"Vogue," Madonna
"Causing a Commotion," Madonna
"Get into the Groove," Madonna
"Rescue Me," Madonna
"Die Another Day," Madonna
"Ride on Time," Black Box
"Everybody," Black Box
"Everybody," C&C Music Factory
"Relax" Frankie Goes to Hollywood"
"Get the Party Started," Pink Featuring Redman
"Do You Want to," Franz Ferdinand
"You Could Be Mine," Guns 'N' Roses
"Welcome to the Jungle," Guns 'N' Roses

"I'm Going to Get You Baby," Bizarre Inc
"Bootylicious," Destiny's Child
"Crazy in Love," Beyoncé
"Love at First Sight," Kylie Monogue
"Can't Get You Outta My Head," Kylie Monogue
"Little Bird," Annie Lennox
"Pride (a Deeper Love)," Aretha Franklin
"Maniac," Flashdance
"Everything to Everyone," Everclear
"I'm Every Woman," Whitney Houston
"Queen of the Night," Whitney Houston
"If I Told You That," Whitney Houston
"If," Janet Jackson
"Escapade," Janet Jackson
"Throb," Janet Jackson
"Rhythm Nation," Janet Jackson
"Nasty," Janet Jackson
"All Nite," Janet Jackson
"Born to be My Baby," Bon Jovi
"All the Small Things," Blink 182
"I Will Follow," U2
"Even Better Than the Real Thing," U2
"Hold Me, Thrill Me, Kiss Me," U2
"I'm Coming out," Diana Ross
"Celebrity Skin," Hole
"Hella Good," No Doubt
"Don't Let Me Down," No Doubt
"Dirty," Christina Aguilera
"Running down a Dream," Tom Petty
"Opportunities," Pet Shop Boys
"100% Pure Love," Crystal Waters
"Superstylin," Groove Armada
"Living on a Prayer," Bon Jovi
"Staying Alive," Bee Gees N-Trance remix
"Mama Said Knock You out," LL Cool J

lower intensity? And is that the most effective way to help lose weight?

The truth is that your body does burn more calories from fat in the "fat burning zone" or at lower intensities but, at higher intensities you burn a greater number of overall calories which is what you should be concerned with when trying to lose weight. Remember, it's very simple, calories in versus calories out, if you burn more calories then you take in you will begin to lose weight. Don't eat a large pepperoni pizza (2,650 cal) and think that doing a half hour of walking the next day will do the trick, because it won't!

It's that simple!

The chart below details the fat calories expended by a 130 pound woman during her cardio session:

What is your Target Heart Rate?

In order to figure out which zone you're in, you first need to know what your target heart rate is. The best way to do this is by using a Karvonen Formula.

Below is an example of the Karvonen formula of a 30-year-old person with a resting heart rate of 60 beats per minute. (To get your resting heart rate, take your pulse for one full minute first thing in the morning.)

220-30 (age) =190
190-60 (resting heart rate) =130
130 x 65% (low end of heart rate) = 84.5 or 130 x 85% (high end) = 110.5
84.5 + 60 (resting heart rate) = 145 OR 110.5 + 60 (rest heart rate) = 171
The target heart rate zone for this person would be 144 to 171

- Climbing stairs is a fantastic way to do cardio and strength training at the same time. To get this 2-in-1 fab workout all you need to do is find a few flights of stairs and climb! Try skipping every other step for 1 minute for every 4 minutes to really work that heart and of course those legs. If you're going to use a Stair-

---

JENNIFER'S MAKE YOU MOVE CD PLAYLIST

Alive 2007, Daft Punk
My Hit Single: "Touch It"

Confessions on a Dance Floor, Madonna
My Hit Singles: "Hung Up," "Sorry," "Get Together," "Jump"

All the Right Reasons, Nickelback
My Hit Singles: "Follow You Home," "Animal," "Rockstar"

Play, Moby
My Hit Single: "Body Rock"

Hysteria, Def Leppard
My Hit Singles: "Pour Some Sugar on Me," "Hysteria"

Slippery When Wet, Bon Jovi
My Hit Singles: "You Give Love a Bad Name," "Living on a Prayer"

Elements of Life, Tiesto
My Hit Singles: I pick all the tracks.

master apply the same principle, go hard for 1 minute then recover at a comfortable pace for 4 minutes. Try doing this 5 times. (Make sure to keep your feet flat on the steps to really feel the burn.)

Tip: Make sure you stand up straight. Only use the rails for balance and not support. This really forces your back and core to work hard too! Besides, the other way is cheating!

In my opinion, the most effective cardio machine is the treadmill. I know you have heard that variety is the key (and it is), but I always go back to the treadmill. As you will see, we can do a million things with it and it is proven to burn the most calories.

Below are five days' worth of treadmill workouts you should try. In my 14-Day Boot Camp, I am asking you to do cardio six times a week for about 30 minutes each time.

The rowing machine gives you a good full-body workout as well, but climbing those stairs is usually more accessible, and my favorite alternative. If you want to try it, the same rule applies, vary your intensity from 1 minute of going as hard as you can, then to a full song at a recovery pace. Repeat five times.

As you will see, on the treadmill, I will switch the amount of time you do and the pace and incline you do it at so your body never relaxes and stops burning as much as it can. Switching it up is key. These high-intensity interval workouts will, unlike basic jogging, increase your resting metabolic rate.

Before starting, always warm up for 5 minutes. A warm-up should be a slow, rhythmic exercise of larger muscle groups done before an activity. This warm-up gets the blood flowing to the muscles and provides the body with a period of adjustment between rest and activity. I use the bike or elliptical machine, when I have access to one, otherwise you can always just walk, or even march, on the spot. Afterwards, make sure you cool down and always stretch. (See the "Cool and the Gang" sidebar.)

Please note that the speed and incline is only a recom-

JENNIFER'S HOT-BODY POWER MOVES SONG PLAYLIST

"Get Off," Prince
"Take Me Out," Franz Ferdinand
"Working for the Weekend," Loverboy
"Animals," Nickleback
"In the Morning," Razorlight
"The Way I Are," Timberland
"I Feel Love," Donna Summer
"Too Funky," George Michael
"The Jump Off," Lil' Kim featuring Mr. Cheeks
"Pour Some Sugar on Me," Def Leppard
"Home Alone," R. Kelly
"That Don't Impress Me Much," Shania Twain
"Lean Back," Fat Joe

mendation and needs to be modified as necessary. This can also by applied without a treadmill by just modifying your pace from slower to faster and vice versa. Inclines are difficult to control when exercising outside, so just do the best you can (which is what this whole book is about!).

Note: In the exercises, you will notice that the incline never goes below 1.5%. This is to simulate the condition of exercising outdoors (wind resistance, road conditions, and varying road grades).

Day 1

For 30–40 minutes, while modifying the speed, walk on an incline. I always start with the highest because I can always go down from there. It's a good motivational trick because your muscles get used to the highest incline and everything from there seems easier. Remember that the lower the incline, the faster the speed. If your treadmill has a 15 incline, start with that and see how well you do. You can always drop. Your starting speed can be 2.2 mph, then work up to 2.8, 3.3 mph, and eventually even faster.

To increase the intensity, hold 3-pound weights.

Day 2

Shock your body by doing a 20-minute run right from the get go. NO more than that! If you would typically start running at 5 miles per hour, do this one at 6.5 miles per hour. Remember to push yourself. You will be surprised at what you can really accomplish! It always seems quite daunting to crank things up as we always start from the same place and only move up incrementally, if at all, so go all out. Also, if you are totally exhausted, you can always decrease it by .5 points, and notch it down to where you need to, but only if you must. And remember, if you start really high, anything lower will seem much easier.

Day 3

Holding light weights, start at a moderate incline of 4 or 5 and walk at a brisk pace of 4.0–4.2 mph for 5 minutes. Then for the next 2 minutes, increase that incline to 12 or so and walk at that same brisk pace. Then take it down to a 1.5 incline and run at 6 mph for 2 minutes then 6.2 mph for 2 minutes, then 6.4 mph for 2 minutes, then 6.6 for 1 minute, and then work it backwards. In other words, then do 6.4 for another 2 minutes, 6.2 for another 2 minutes, and then 6.0 for another 2 minutes. Then increase the incline back to 4 and run at a slower pace of 5.0 for 5 minutes. Reduce the incline to 1.5 and jog at a pace of 6.0 for 2 minutes, then, increase the incline to 4 at the same pace for 1 minute, then drop the speed completely to about 3.5 mph for another minute. This is a little complicated, but it's worth it for the intensity alone.

Day 4

On this day we're adding something new to the mix altogether. Now it might sound scary to the total beginner, but trust me, once you get used to it, you will be a pro. I'm referring to walking and sometimes jogging backwards on the treadmill. This is my favorite and it really works the opposing muscle groups, and guards against muscle imbalance. At the beginning you can take it slowly and even hold onto the side railings, but once you gain your balance, slowly remove your hands. This also requires you to use your balance and stabilizing muscle groups, which I always try to incorporate into every one of my exercises. Start walking briskly for a few minutes and then turn around and walk backwards for 2 minutes (with this go at your own pace and work up slowly). Try 2.5–3.0 mph and move up. Then walk, jog, or run for 5 minutes the normal way and then go backwards for 2 minutes again. Remember, the more comfortable you get, the faster you will be able to go. Do this routine for 30 minutes.

Day 5

Go from 30 seconds of running as fast as you can to 2 minutes of walking briskly. Repeat this between 8-10 times on a 1.5 incline. The last 5 minutes should be used to challenge all different angles of your muscles. You will do this by slowing the speed between 2.5-3.5 mph. Skip for 30 seconds, walk backwards for 30 seconds, forward for 30 seconds, stand sideways and shuffle with your right foot leading for 30 seconds, walk for 30 seconds forwards, and then repeat with the left foot leading for 30 seconds.

Now as you get more familiar with the guidelines, you will be able to tweak this program and mix it up a bit. Also, when doing such an intense cardio program, make sure you get a lot of stabilizing exercises and stretching work in. A yoga or Pilates class, or a couple of laps at your local swimming pool, once or twice a week will balance things out nicely.

COOL AND THE GANG

Cooling down can be just simply walking or marching on the spot for a few minutes to lower your heart rate. Stretching, though, is a great way to cool down, and as flexibility exercises are a key component of a balanced fitness program (it protects against injury), you have a double act. There are many schools of thought on stretching, but most fitness experts agree that the following principles are the safest and most effective. After you exercise, your cool-down and stretch should last between 5–10 minutes.

1. Use static stretching. Static stretching involves a slow, gradual, and controlled elongation of a muscle through its full range of motion, held for 15–30 seconds in the furthest comfortable position without pain. In my opinion, all stretches for each muscle group should be done by using this static form of stretching.

2. Stretch daily. Daily stretching is best during, and after exercise sessions. Frequent stretching will help you avoid muscular imbalances, knots, tightness, and muscle soreness.

3. Always warm up before stretching. Never stretch a cold muscle! It's dangerous. As I said, warming up gets blood circulating throughout the body and into the muscles, and a warm muscle is much more easily and safely stretched than a cold one. Your warm-up should last about 5 minutes and should be similar to the activity that you are about to do, but at a much lower intensity.

THE STRETCH SET

Your key limber-up, loosen-up moves from top to bottom:

1. Cross Shoulder Stretch

Stand up straight, with knees slightly bent. Place feet hip distance apart, making sure your toes are pointing forward. Keeping your shoulders even, bend your right arm at the elbow joint, extending your arm across your chest. Place your left hand on the right elbow to gently support the arm during this stretch. Feel it in your right arm and shoulder. Inhale through your nose, and exhale through your mouth as you complete this stretch. Hold it for a count of eight. Repeat this stretch on the opposite side, using your right hand to stretch the left arm and shoulder.

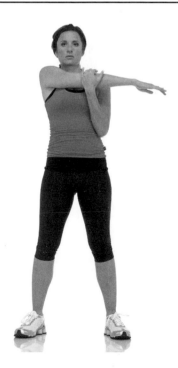

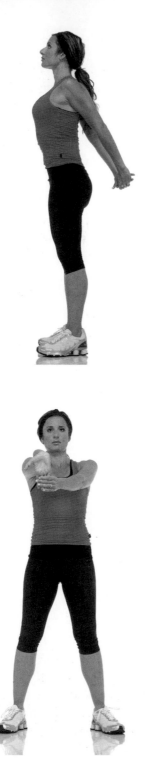

2. Chest Stretch

Stand up straight, with knees slightly bent. Place your feet hip distance apart, making sure your toes are pointing forward. Keeping your shoulders even, place your arms behind your back. Clasp your hands together and extend your arms out. Hold this position for the count of 8. Feel the stretch in your chest. Inhale through your nose, and exhale through your mouth as you complete this stretch.

3. Bicep Stretch

Stand up straight, with knees slightly bent. Place your feet hip distance apart, making sure your toes are pointing forward. Keeping your shoulders even, extend your right arm out in front of you, palm facing up, and bend your fingers back slightly. Feel a gentle stretch in your forearm and bicep muscles. Hold stretch for a count of 8. Repeat the stretch on the opposite side using your left arm.

4. Tricep Stretch

Stand up straight, with knees slightly bent. Place your feet hip distance apart, making sure your toes are pointing forward. Keeping your shoulders even as you complete this stretch, bend your right arm at the elbow while lifting your arm next to your head. Position your right fingers so they touch the shoulder blade area. At the same time, place your left arm across the top of your head, and place your left hand on the right elbow to gently support the arm during this stretch. Feel the stretch in your right tricep. Inhale through your nose, and exhale through your mouth as you complete this stretch. Hold stretch for a count of 8. Repeat this stretch on the opposite side using your right hand to support your left arm while stretching your left tricep.

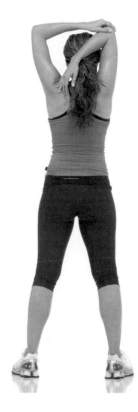

5. Groin Stretch

Sit with your feet together, your head up, and your elbows positioned on the inside of your knees. Then slowly push down on the inside of your knees with your elbows. You should feel the stretch along the inside of your thighs. Hold the stretch for 10 to 15 seconds. Repeat 5 times.

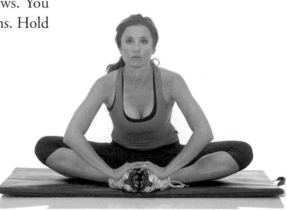

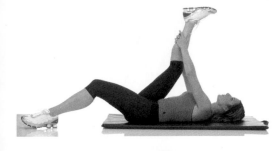

6. Hamstring Stretch

Lie down with your back flat on your mat, with both of your knees bent. Place your feet flat on the floor, about 6 inches apart. Bend your right knee up to your chest and hold onto your right thigh with both hands placed behind your knee. Slowly straighten your right leg, feeling the slight stretching in the back of your leg. Hold the stretch for 20 seconds, and then repeat the stretch with your left leg.

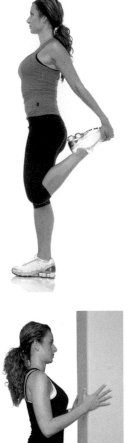

7. Quad Stretch

Stand facing a wall, about 1 foot away from it. Balance yourself by putting your right hand against the wall. Raise your right leg behind you and grab your foot with your left hand. Pull your heel gently up toward your bottom, stretching the muscles in the front of your right thigh for 20 seconds. Keep your thighs close together to keep your knee aligned and the stretch effective. Repeat the stretch with your left leg.

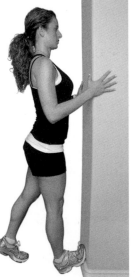

8. Calf Stretch

Stand facing a wall, about 2 feet away from it. Keeping your heels flat and your back straight, lean forward and press your hands and forehead to the wall. Make sure your knees do not move forward over your ankles. Do this slowly. You should feel the stretch in the muscles in the back of your lower legs, above your heels. If you need a bigger stretch, move farther away from the wall. Hold this position for 20 seconds and then relax. Repeat.

PART 2: POWER MOVES

Now it's time to learn the Power Moves, exercises that will give you maximum results in the minimum amount of time. I guarantee that they will ROCK your body into shape.

Part of my back-to-basics philosophy is that there is "no gym required!" Yes, you read that correctly! NO… GYM … REQUIRED.

With the Power Moves I'll give you here, you will be literally tapping into your own power, using the power of your own body weight as resistance, to get into shape. (And research also shows that weight-bearing exercise strengthens the bones as well.) So now we've completely eliminated the "I don't have time to get to the gym" excuse.

In fact, with a very basic tool kit outlined below (which includes *you* as the main tool—remember, you're the lead singer in this band), you can do these exercises or their variations just about anywhere—at home, in a hotel, garden, park, or on the beach. If you do enjoy going to the gym, of course, that works too. The point is you don't have to be a member at a gym, and even if you are and happen to be out of town or unable to make it, you can pretty much perform these Power Moves wherever you happen to be. That is, your "stage" can be anywhere.

NO GYM REQUIRED: YOUR BASIC TOOL KIT

1. Swiss Exercise ball: Make sure you order the right size for your height:
   5 feet 3 inches and shorter = 55 centimeters
   5 feet 4 inches–5 feet 10 inches = 65 centimeters
   5 feet 11 inches and taller = 75 centimeters

2. Medicine ball
3. Mat
4. Free weights/adjustable weight system: They go from 2.5 pounds to 15 pounds.

Remember that with weights you need to keep challenging yourself. If you can do an entire set of 12–15 repetitions easily, you should increase the weight.

5. Skipping rope (a weighted skipping rope is a great option too)
6. A chair
7. A platform/step
8. Stop watch
9. Heart rate monitor: You want to maintain a heart rate that is between 70–80% percent of your maximum heart rate.

---

10. Exercise tubing: These come in several levels of difficulty. You may want to have two or three on hand in order to increase your resistance.

11. Xerdisc: This circular piece of plastic can be used for balanced training and stability work for both upper and lower body conditioning. It's not a mandatory tool but it can help improve balance and stability. Try standing on one foot for 30 seconds then switch as a good basic exercise. This will also strengthen your ankles.

12. NGR fitness shoes: These come with interchangeable weighted insoles that allow you to increase resistance as you get more fit. Remember ankle weights? These have the same concept but the weight is distributed evenly on your sole which is way better for your joints. You can wear them just doing your errands or when working out to really increase that calorie burn and resistance. Check out www.nogymrequired.com to see where you can pick up a pair.

To make it easy to identify which tool(s) you'll use for which exercise, next to each of the Power Moves, you'll see the corresponding symbols of the tools required as shown above.

Of course, you won't have to use all of these tools at once. You may not necessarily have access to some of the tools if you're traveling, for example. But, fear not. I have created variations for many of the exercises as well. Again, there's no excuse not to work out anymore when there's a "no gym required." Solution: If you're on the road (like Rock Stars often are), you really only need to take a resistance band and a skipping rope—both of these are easy to pack!

Like the Rock Star who gives it her all, you are going to sweat! I promise you that with these Power Moves. They're designed to be multifunctional; that is, you'll always work more than one body part at a time—that's how you gain efficiency in time spent and gain maximum impact.

The Power Moves will focus heavily on engaging your core—the true "rock" in your "star" body. I call it the ABC principle: it's All aBout the Core. All of these exercises involve working on your core strength, and they will not only test, but also help improve your balance, stability, and flexibility. Yes, indeed, they will give you the toned-up, defined look every Rock Star needs for her daily appearances on the "stage" of life.

You'll notice that each of the Power Moves is also rated as Gold, Platinum, or Double Platinum.

• Gold is a Level 1 exercise
• Platinum is a Level 2 exercise
• Double Platinum is a Level 3 exercise

You can mix and match these moves according to the level you feel most comfortable at to work the various body parts. With each exercise description, you'll also notice that the muscle groups engaged are specified: Abs, butt (glutes), hamstrings, quads, thighs, calves, biceps, triceps, deltoids, and, of course, your heart—yes, you'll work them all.

There's nothing more frustrating than reading about an exercise and trying to figure out how it is supposed to be performed when there are only words and no photos. So, you'll notice there are lots of photos here—one for every move, in fact. Just like you'll visualize yourself as being in Rock Star shape from the outset, these photos are here to help you visualize how you'll perform each move.

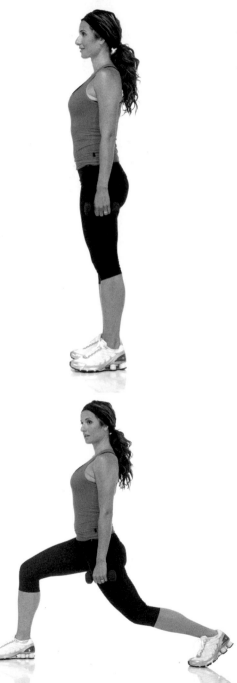

You've Got the Power With My Fab 40 Hot-Body Power Moves

1. Walking Lunges

- *How to:* With a 5- to 8-pound free weight in each hand, start with feet together, and step forward with one leg out, bending the knee at a right angle, not quite touching the ground. Alternate legs and continue across a distance of at least 30 feet. Do not extend the knee forward past the ankle. This puts excessive and unnecessary strain on the knee. As an added benefit, lunges not only work the entire set of glutes, but it will develop a more beautifully defined pair of legs too.

  - *Rock Star muscle groups:* Quads, glutes, hamstrings, abs/core

  - *Basic tools:* Free weights

  - *Repetitions per set:* Length of room (3 sets). Try for a minimum of 10.

  - *Level:* Gold

  - *Variation:* If you don't have enough space, i.e., you're in a hotel room, eliminate the walking element and lunge on the spot.

2. Walking Lunges with Twist

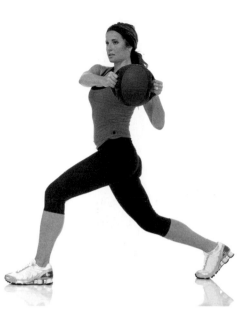

- *How to:* Same as above, but drop the free weights and use a medicine ball instead. With each lunge, extend the medicine ball in front of you, and twist in the direction toward the leg that is extended forward.

  - *Rock Star muscle groups:* Quads, hamstrings, abs/core (obliques)

  - *Basic tool:* Medicine ball

  - *Repetitions per set:* Length of room (3 sets). Minimum of 10 per set.

  - *Level:* Platinum

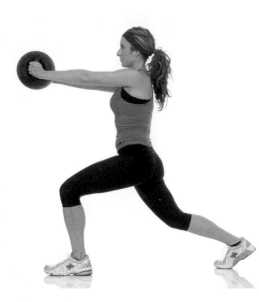

3. Reverse Lunge with Medicine Ball

- *How to:* With arms extended, hold a medicine ball at shoulder height, then lunge backwards, making sure your knees are bent at a 90-degree angle. Alternating legs after every rep

  - *Rock Star muscle groups:* Quads, glutes, hamstrings, and hip flexors

  - *Basic tool:* Medicine ball or free weight

  - *Repetitions per set:* 15–20 (3 sets)

  - *Level:* Platinum

  - *Variation:* To increase the difficulty of this move, lunge off the back of a step platform.

4. Bulgarian Lunge

- *How to:*
  - Begin by standing about 3 feet in front of a platform (your back toward the bench), hands on hips (*beginning*) or holding dumbbells (*advanced*).
  - Place your right foot on the bench, insuring your left leg is still straight in alignment with your upper body (if not, adjust your foot placement).
  - Slowly descend, just like in a regular lunge—remembering to keep your left knee behind your left foot (your target depth is where your left leg is in a 90 degree bend position).
  - Hold for 2 seconds, then extend your left leg and return to the beginning position.

    - *Rock Star muscle groups:* Glutes, hamstrings, quads, calves, and hip flexors

    - *Basic tools:* Step (platform), or a stack of books/magazines

    - *Repetitions per set:* 12–15 per leg (3 sets)

    - *Level:* Gold

    - *Variation:* Hold heavy free weights in your hands to increase intensity.

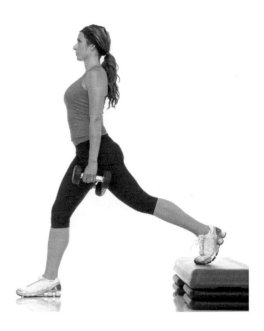

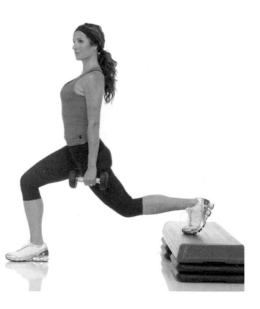

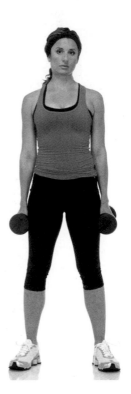

5. Crossover Lunge with Hammer Curl

- *How to:* Stand with your feet hip-width apart. Step your right foot diagonally forward and across the left foot. Slowly lower your left knee until the right leg is parallel to the floor. Then using the right leg, push yourself back into starting position. Repeat the same motion with the left leg.

  - *Rock Star muscle groups:* Quads, outer thighs, calves, and hamstrings

  - *Basic tools:* Free weights

  - *Repetitions per set:* 12–15 per leg (3 sets)

  - *Level:* Platinum

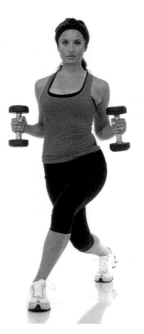

6. Wall Squat Plus 21s

- *How to:* Place an exercise ball between your lower back and the wall while holding a dumbbell in each hand. Slowly lower your body, rolling the ball down the wall with the small of your back until your thighs are parallel to the ground. While you are holding this position, you will do a super set of bicep curls. Curl until elbows hit 90 degrees, then lower to the starting position. Do 7 reps. Follow immediately with another 7 reps, this time bringing your dumbbells to your armpits, then lowering until your elbows reach 90 degrees. Finish with 7 complete curls, lowering your dumbbells to your hips and curling them all the way back up. Keep holding that squat for another count of 21 then roll the ball back up to starting position.

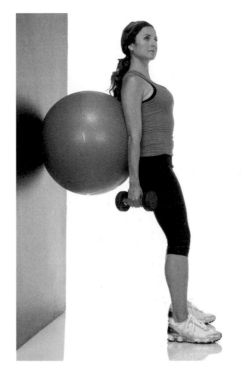

  - *Rock Star muscle groups:* Butt, quads, hamstrings, abs/core (lower back), and biceps

  - *Basic tools:* Exercise ball and free weights

  - *Repetitions per set:* 21

  - *Level:* Platinum; to make this a Gold-level exercise, only squat down half the way down.

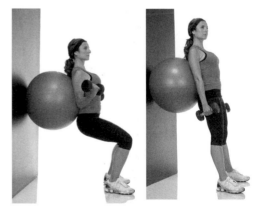

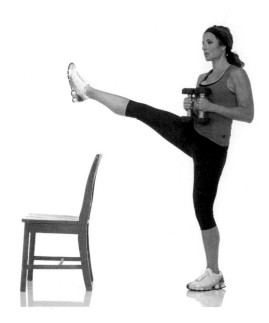

7. Swing Kick

- *How to:* With a chair in front of you, stand with two feet together, holding free weights steady at the centre of your chest. Lift right leg counterclockwise in a swinging motion over the back of the chair. Follow by lifting left leg in a swinging motion clockwise over the back of the chair. Repeat, alternating each leg.

  - *Rock Star muscle groups:* Outer thighs, hip flexors, abs/core

  - *Basic tools:* Free weights, chair

  - *Repetitions per set:* 20–25 (3 sets)

  - *Level:* Platinum; to make this a Gold-level exercise, eliminate the free weights and do only 2 sets.

8. Standing Side Crunch

- *How to:* Stand with feet a little more than hip distance apart. With a free weight in each hand, raise your right arm up in an arc over your head and then down while lifting your right knee up toward the side of your body to meet your right elbow . Repeat on the left side.

  - *Rock Star muscle groups:* Abs/core (obliques, glutes, deltoids)

  - *Basic tools:* Free weights

  - *Repetitions per set:* 12–15 per side (3 sets)

  - *Level:* Platinum/Double Platinum (with heavier weights); to make this a Gold-level move, eliminate the free weights.

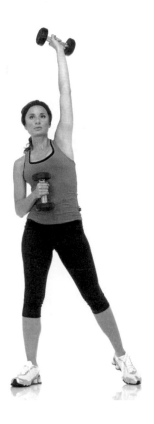

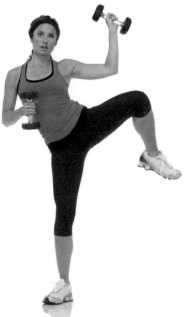

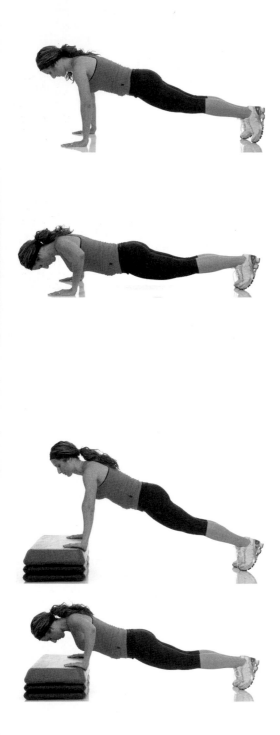

9. Push-ups

- *How to:* Lie face down with your legs straight out behind you and your feet together. Position your palms so they are directly under your elbows. When your arms are bent, they should form a 90-degree angle. Your neck should be straight and your eyes should be focused on the floor in front of you. Keep your abs tight. Straighten your arms so that your body is hovering over the floor, balancing on your palms and the balls of your feet. Now, bend elbows and lower your entire body at once until your upper arms are parallel with the floor, exhale, then push back up to the starting position. Repeat.

- *Rock Star muscle groups:* Abs/core, chest, triceps, shoulders, and back

- *Basic tool:* Just you

- *Repetitions per set:* 10 (3 sets)

- *Level:* Gold; to make this Platinum, add 10 more consecutively to each set

- *Variation:* If this is too difficult, begin using a bench and place your palms several inches wider than shoulder-width apart. Try and avoid doing "girl" push-ups on your hands and knees. This version is better because it still forces you to engage your core muscles, whereas the "girl" version does not.

10. Push-ups with Exercise Ball

- *How to:* See previous and then modify it by placing your ankles on an exercise ball and your palms on the floor. This really works your core and stabilizing muscle groups, not to mention it's a fantastic move to hone your balance.

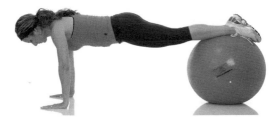

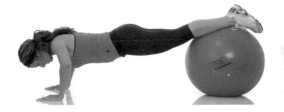

  - *Rock Star muscle groups:* Abs/core, chest, triceps, hamstrings, shoulders

  - *Basic tools:* Exercise ball

  - *Repetitions per set:* 10–12 (3 sets)

  - *Level:* Double Platinum

  - *Variation:* Place toes on a step platform instead and this will become an intermediate move.

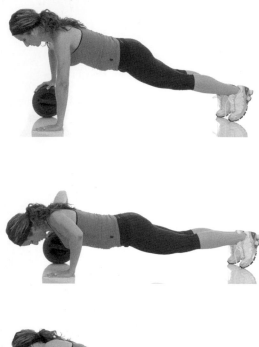

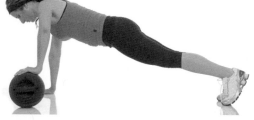

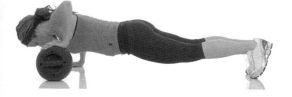

11. One-handed Walkover Push-ups

- *How to:* Start in a push-up position, with your left hand on the ball and you're your right hand on the floor, and do a pushup. At the top of the exercise, roll the ball, and place your right hand on the ball, with your left hand on the floor, and do another push-up. Repeat.

  - *Rock Star muscle groups:* Abs/core, chest triceps, quads, shoulders

  - *Basic tools:* Medicine ball

  - *Repetitions per set:* 8–10

  - *Level:* Double Platinum

  - *Variation:* For walking push-ups, you don't need a medicine ball. After every push-up, walk your *hands and toes out a few inch*es, then do another push-up. Do this until you get to the other side of the room.

12. Alternating Arm Shoulder Press on Exercise Ball

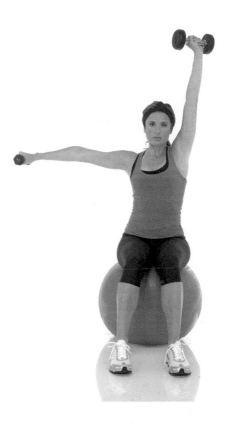

- *How to:* Sit down on the ball. Press your right arm up with your heavier-weight (usually 8 lbs) dumbbell for 10 reps. While doing this, extend the other arm out to the side at shoulder level while holding your lightest weight. Switch arms after every set. You should do one set of 10 on each arm, a second set of 8, and a third set of 6.

  - *Rock Star muscle groups:* Shoulders, abs/core.

  - *Basic tools:* Exercise ball, free weights

  - *Repetitions per set:* 10, 8, 6 (3 sets)

  - *Level:* Gold

  - *Variation:* To make this a Platinum exercise, increase the weight and lift one foot a few inches off the ground, then switch feet for next set.

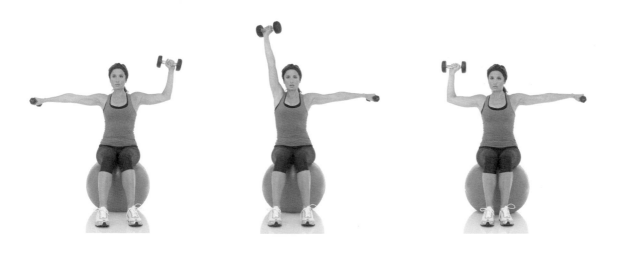

13. Chest Press on Ball and Crunch

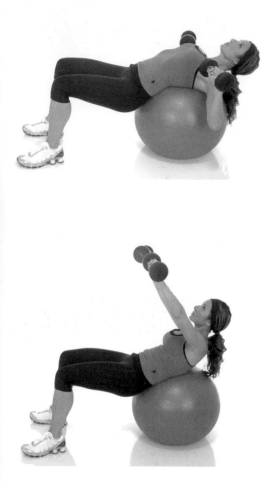

- *How to:* Lie down on the ball with your lower back and neck on the ball. Both legs should be planted firmly on the ground at a 90 degree angle. Your torso should be parallel to the floor. Keeping your butt raised, bend the elbows and lower the arms down until the elbows are just below the chest (arms should look like goal posts). Press the weights up while you exhale without locking the elbows. Do a crunch at the same time.

  - *Rock Star muscle groups:* Chest, core, butt

  - *Basic tools:* Exercise ball, weights

  - *Repetitions per set:* 12–15 (3 sets)

  - *Level:* Gold

  - *Variation:* To make this a Platinum exercise, increase the weight and/or try lifting one leg a few inches off the ground during each rep. Alternate legs.

14. Lying Leg Crossovers, "Scissor Sisters"

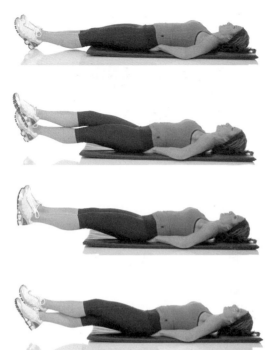

- *How to:* Lie down on your mat with your hands under your lower back, elbows bent. Raise your legs in a V-formation about 4 inches off the mat and cross your right leg over to the right and then over the left leg in smooth controlled succession.

  - *Rock Star muscle groups:* Abs/core (lower abs, outer thighs)

  - *Basic tool:* Mat

  - *Repetitions per set:* 12–15

  - *Level:* Gold

  - *Variation:* If you have any lower back pain, the bicycle crunch is a great alternative:

    1. Lie face up on the floor and lace your fingers behind your head.

    2. Bring the knees in towards the chest and lift the shoulder blades off the ground without pulling on the neck.

    3. Straighten the left leg out to about a 45-degree angle while simultaneously turning the upper body to the right, bringing the left elbow towards the right knee.

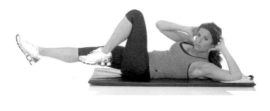

    4. Switch sides, bringing the right elbow towards the left knee.

    5. Continue alternating sides.

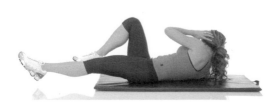

15. Exercise Ball Crunch

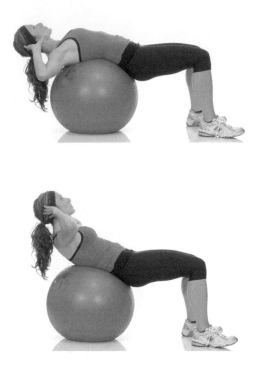

- *How to:* Sit on a Swiss ball with your feet hip width apart on the floor. Put your hands behind your head, elbows out, and your eyes and chin up. Slowly pull your abs inward as you lean back and your entire back and shoulders are resting on the ball. Exhale as you crunch up until your shoulder blades are off the ball completely. Hold for a second and then inhale as you slowly lower back down.

- *Rock star muscle groups:* Abs/core

- *Basic tool:* Swiss ball

- *Repetitions per set:* 20

- *Level:* Gold

- *Variation:* You can also challenge yourself further by performing this exact exercise with one foot hovering a few inches off the floor. This forces your hip stabilizer and abs to work even harder to keep you balanced throughout the movement. Doing a crunch on the ball is way more effective than the ground because it allows for a fuller range of motion and develops core stability.

16. Back Extension on Ball

- *How to:* If you're a beginner, prop the ball against something sturdy like a wall for added stability. Position the ball under your hips and lower torso with the knees straight or bent. With hands behind the head or back, slowly roll down the ball. Lift your chest off the ball, bringing your shoulders up until your body is in a straight line. Make sure your body is in alignment (i.e., head, neck, shoulders, and back are in a straight line), your abs are pulled in and don't hyperextend the back.

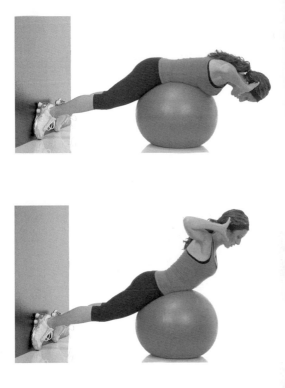

- *Rock Star muscle groups:* Lower back, abs/core

- *Basic tool:* Exercise ball

- *Repetitions per set:* 12–15 (3 sets)

- *Level:* Gold; to make this a Platinum-level exercise, extend your arms directly in front of you with your elbows aligned with your ears. Also, you can get rid of the wall for that added support.

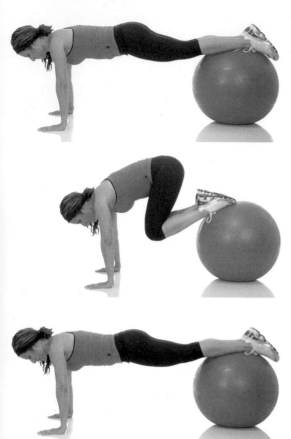

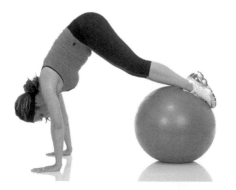

17. Swiss Ball Leg Pull-in

- *How to:* Place feet with toes down onto the exercise ball while extending your body out from the ball and assuming a push-up position. Slowly move ball in and out in a steady, controlled motion using the front portion of your feet.

  - *Rock Star muscle groups:* Abs/core, hamstrings, quads, shoulders

  - *Basic tool:* Swiss ball

  - *Repetitions per set:* 12–15

  - *Level:* Platinum

  - *Variation:* Assume the pike position on the way in with the ball and this becomes a Double Platinum exercise. (For this, keep the legs straight, contract the abs and pull the ball in a pike position until toes are on the ball.)

18. Lying Down Ball Raises

- *How to:* Lie down flat on your mat with an exercise ball between your ankles. Raise and lower your legs (ball stabilized between them) in a controlled motion without allowing the ball to ever touch the mat.

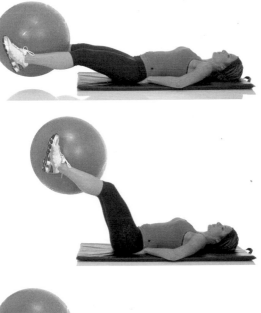

  - *Rock Star muscle groups:* Abs/core, hip flexors, inner and outer thighs

  - *Basic tools:* Mat, exercise ball

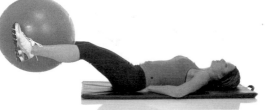

  - *Repetitions per set:* 12–15 (3 sets)

  - *Level:* Gold

  - *Variation:* To make this Platinum, on your last rep, hover the ball 4 inches off the floor and squeeze your inner thighs together for a count of 8 a few times. This is a great one to target those inner thighs and burn your abs.

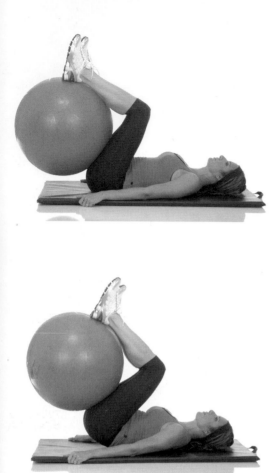

19. Reverse Crunch with Ball

- *How to:* There are many ways to do reverse crunches, but one of the best is to put an exercise ball under your knees. Make sure you contract your abs and use them to lift your hips off the floor. It's a very small movement and you shouldn't swing or use momentum.

  - *Rock Star muscle groups:* Abs/core

  - *Basic tool:* Exercise ball

  - *Repetitions per set:* 12–15

  - *Level:* Platinum

  - *Variation:* Legs raised with no ball and pulse up.

20. Side-Lying Triangle with Ball

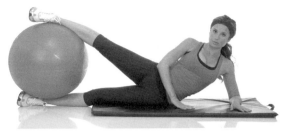

- *How to:* Lie on your right side with a stability ball between your legs by your ankles, hips stacked on top of each other and the right elbow on the floor. Push yourself up to your right hand and hold. Lift your left arm so it's in line with your left shoulder. Twist your upper body toward the floor and reach your left arm underneath your body. Return to starting position and repeat. Switch sides.

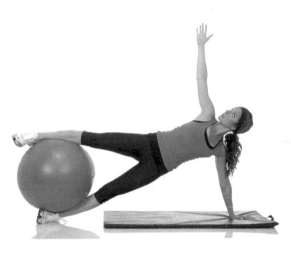

  - *Rock Star muscle groups:* Abs/core, obliques, inner and outer thighs, shoulders

  - *Basic tool:* Excercise ball

  - *Repetitions per set:* 12–15

  - *Level:* Double Platinum

  - *Variation:* No ball makes this a Gold level.

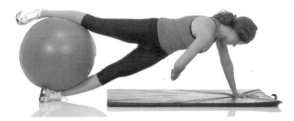

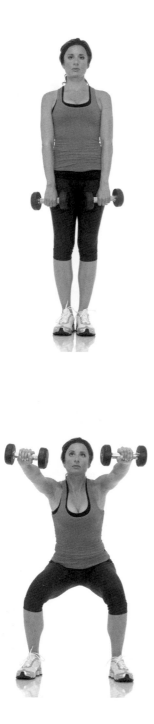

23. Lateral Squat with or without Resistant Band

- *How to*: Stand with your feet shoulder-width apart. Start by stepping to the right with your right foot and proceed into a squat. Return to the standing position with your feet shoulder width apart. Now step to your left with your left foot and proceed into a squat. Return to the starting position and repeat.

  - *Rock Star muscle groups*: Outer thighs, glutes, quads

  - *Basic tool(s)*: resistant band (optional)

  - *Repetitions per set*: 15

  - *Level*: Gold

  - *Variations*: Tie a resistant band around your ankles when doing this move and it becomes a platinum move. This will also engage your stabilizing muscles. You can also add a shoulder press if you want to include your upper body.

24. Lateral lunge with Shoulder Raise

- *How to:* Stand with your feet hip-width apart, arms at your sides and a dumbbell in each hand. Step your right leg out to the side about a stride's length, keeping your right foot parallel to your left foot. Lean onto your right leg, bending at the hip, until your right thigh is parallel to the floor. As you are lowering yourself into a lunge, simultaneously raise the dumbbells up in front of you to eye level with palms facing down. Then, using the right leg, exhale and push yourself back into the starting position. Repeat with the left leg.

  - *Rock Star muscle groups:* Butt, quads, hamstrings, abs/core, shoulders

  - *Basic tools:* Free weights, step platform (optional)

  - *Repetitions per set:* 12–15 (3 sets)

  - *Level:* Platinum

  - *Variations:* No shoulder raise will make it Gold.

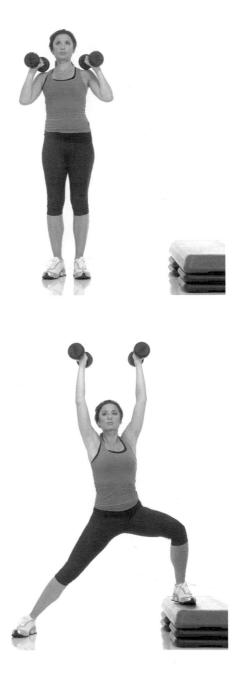

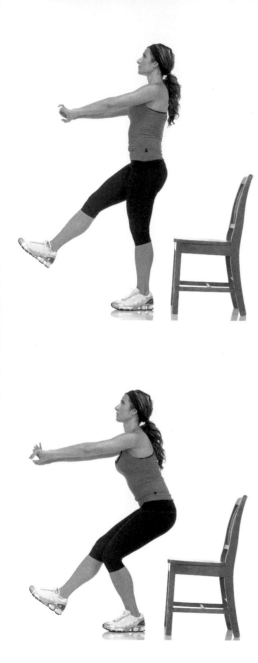

25. One-Leg Squat

- *How to:* Place a bench directly behind you (just in case you wipe out). Stand on your right leg. Lift your left foot a couple of inches off the ground. The basic moves of a squat apply here. Keep your abs tight and your heel on the ground. Be careful not to lean forward or to let your knee move beyond your toes. Slowly lower yourself down until your glutes barely tap the bench, exhale, and stand up straight on the right leg only. Continue for a full set on the right leg and then switch over to the left.

- *Rock Star muscle groups:* Glutes, quads, hamstrings, core muscles

- *Basic tool:* Bench/chair

- *Repetitions per set:* 8–10 (3 sets)

- *Level:* Platinum

- *Variation:* To make this Gold, try this move with your lower back pressed on an exercise ball against a wall. This gives you a lot more support and stability.

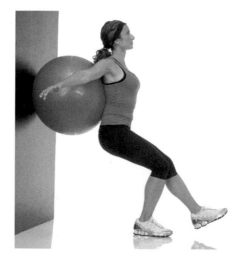

26. Jumping Jack Squats

- *How to:* With your arms over your head, spread your feet out while bending your knees and keeping your weight on the balls of your feet. Bounce twice with feet spread apart, then bring the feet back together, bouncing twice again. Repeat complete jacks, out and in.

  - *Rock Star muscle groups:* Butt, quads, hamstrings, abs/core (obliques, adductors)

  - *Basic tool(s):* Just you or with light weights

  - *Repetitions per set:* 15 (3 sets)

  - *Level:* Gold; make this Platinum by adding free weights.

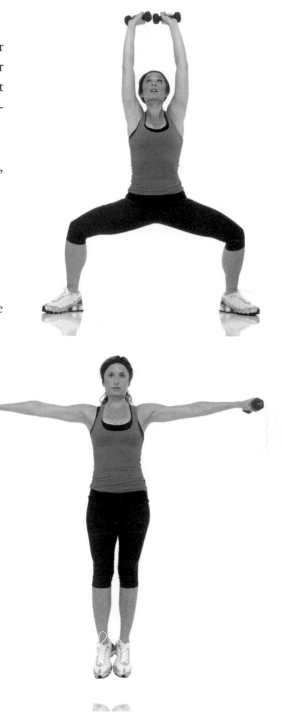

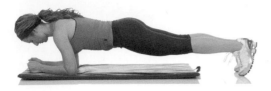

27. Basic Plank

- *How to:* Lie face down on your mat. Raise up on to your elbows and your toes, ensuring your hips are raised to make your body a parallel "plank." Squeeze abs and butt while doing this and hold for as long as you can.

  - *Rock Star muscle groups:* Abs/core, hamstrings, butt, quads, shoulders

  - *Basic tools:* Mat

  - *Repetitions per set:* Try for 30 seconds and work your way up from there

  - *Level:* Gold

  - *Variation:* Plank with twist (Platinum), plank leg out (Platinum), plank tower (Double Platinum)

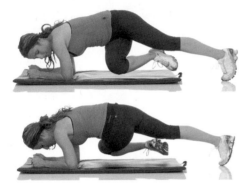

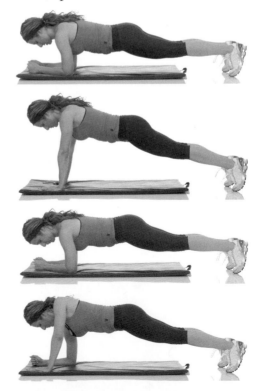

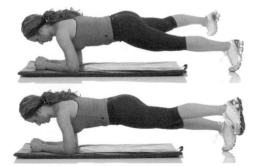

28. Plank on Exercise Ball

- *How to:* On your knees place your elbows on the ball and roll forward a bit until your back is flat. Then straighten your knees and hold into a plank position for 30 seconds.
  See previous for other details.

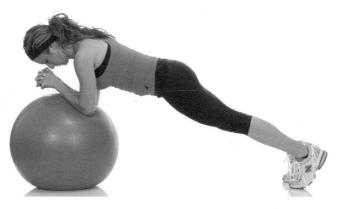

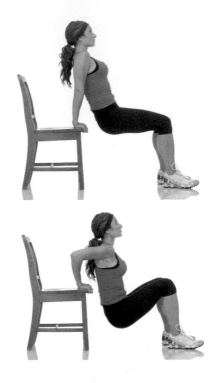

29. Tricep Dips

- *How to:* Stand with your back to a sturdy bench or chair. Bend your legs as if to sit and place your palms on the front edge about shoulder-width apart. Position your feet in front of you so that most of your body weight is resting on your arms. Keeping your elbows tucked along your sides, inhale and bend your arms. Slowly lower your body until your upper arms are parallel to the floor. Your hips should drop straight down toward the ground, always staying as close to the bench as possible. Hold for a second, then exhale and straighten your arms back to the starting position. Be careful not to lower your body too far or you will overstress your shoulders. Do not lean forward or away from the bench, which also creates stress on your shoulders.

- *Rock Star muscle groups:* Triceps, shoulders, chest

- *Basic tool:* Chair or bench

- *Repetitions per set:* 12–15 (3 sets)

- *Level:* Gold

- *Variation:* Straighten your legs in front of you with your heels pressed into the ground; or to make it even harder, use an exercise ball instead of a bench or chair. Another option is even to place your lower legs on a Swiss ball while your hands are on the bench/chair and dip down that way.

30. One-Handed Tricep Dips with One-Leg out

- *How to:* This is one of my favorites! The basic moves of a tricep dip apply here (see previous), but extend your right foot out in front of you and take the opposite hand off the bench, then dip slowly. Continue the full set and switch sides.

  - *Rock Star muscle groups:* Abs/core, triceps, butt, quads, hamstrings; also great for coordination and balance

  - *Basic tools:* Platform, step, stack of books/magazines, or chair

  - *Repetitions per set:* 8–10 (3 sets)

  - *Level:* Double Platinum

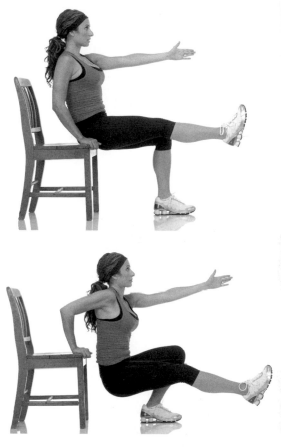

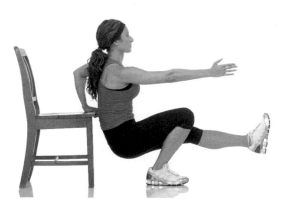

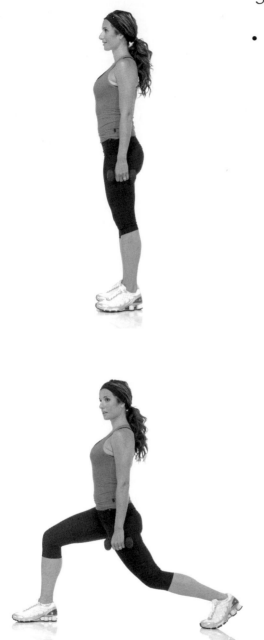

31. Lunge 10 Hut (10:1 and back)

- *How to:* See Walking Lunge (earlier) for starting position. With a 5–8-pound free weight in each hand, start with your feet together, and step forward with one leg out, bending the knee to a right angle, not quite touching the ground. On your first step out, you will pulse (lift and lower) for a count of 1, then alternate legs for a pulse of 2 and so on until you get to 10. On the way back, you will start with the opposite leg and pulse for 10 and alternate the leg for a pulse of 9, and so on until you get back down to 1. This is a KILLER!

  - *Rock Star muscle groups:* Quads, glutes, hamstrings and calves

  - *Basic tools:* Free weights

  - *Repetitions per set:* Length of room (3 sets);

  - *Level:* Platinum

  - *Variation:* If you're a beginner, go up to 6 and back to 1. Work up to 10!

32. Leg Curl with Swiss Ball

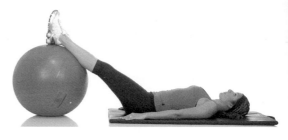

- *How to:* Lie down flat on your mat with both feet on top of an exercise ball. Raise your butt off the mat and then begin rolling the exercise ball in toward your butt and back out.

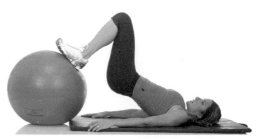

  - *Rock Star muscle groups:* Abs/core, hamstrings, glutes

  - *Basic tools:* Exercise ball, mat

  - *Repetitions per set:* 12–15

  - *Level:* Gold;

  - *Variation:* To make this a Double Platinum exercise, do a Single Leg Curl by placing one leg on the ball while raising the other in the air and then move the ball in toward your butt and back out with the one leg. Alternate leg each rep.

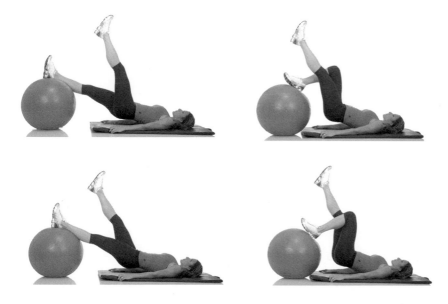

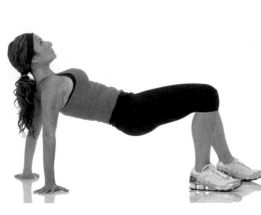

33. Crab Walk

- *How to:* Face up, lower your body into a supine position, with your hands out to your sides about 10 inches from your shoulders. Push yourself into a "crab" or "bridge" position. Your legs should be bent with feet positioned just below your knees. Walk forward then backwards in this position for as many steps as you can without falling.

  - *Rock Star muscle groups:* Shoulders, back, glutes, triceps

  - *Basic tool:* Just you

  - *Repetitions per set:* From one side of the room and back

  - *Level:* Gold

34. Stationary Boxing Jabs Using Dumbbells

- *How to:* Simply stand with feet shoulder-width apart and with one foot slightly more forward than the other. With your fists positioned in front of your chin and holding 3-pound weights, start punching forward while twisting at your waist. Increase the length of time you can do this between other exercises. The heavier the weight and the longer the duration, the greater the level of intensity.

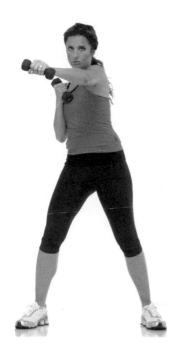

  - *Rock Star muscle groups:* Arms, obliques, abs, core, back

  - *Basic tool:* Free weights

  - *Repetitions per set:* 30 seconds to start and you can move up from there.

  - *Level:* Gold/ Platinum

  - *Variation:* Do exercise with no weights.

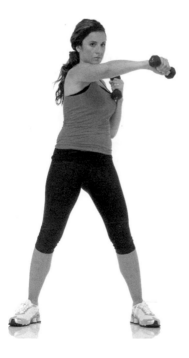

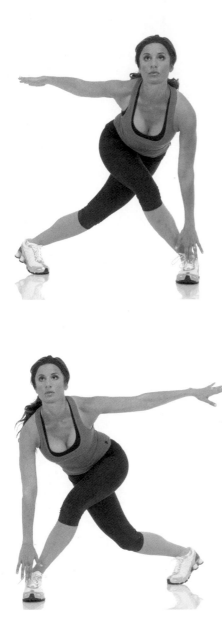

35. Speed Skating

- *How to:* Stand hip-width apart and bend from the waist. Put weight on your right leg, keeping your right knee slightly bent and your abs pulling in. Swing your arm to the right, now push off your right foot, shifting your body weight and your arms to the left. Repeat this skater-like motion for 30 seconds and work your way up to 1 minute and so on.

  - *Rock star muscle groups:* Total lower body and your heart

  - *Basic tool:* You

  - *Repetition per set:* 30 seconds to start start and work your way up to 1 minute

  - *Level:* Gold

  - *Variation:* Hold light weights in your hands to add some upper body resistance.

36. Bicep Curls with Resistant Band

- *How to:* Stand on the band and hold handles with palms facing out. Keeping abs in and knees slightly bent, bend arms and bring palms toward shoulders in a bicep curl. Position feet wider for more tension. Return to start and repeat.

  - *Rock star muscle groups:* Biceps

  - *Basic tool:* Resistant band

  - *Repetition per set:* 15

  - *Level:* Gold

  - *Variation:* Move your arm out to the side to work a different angle.

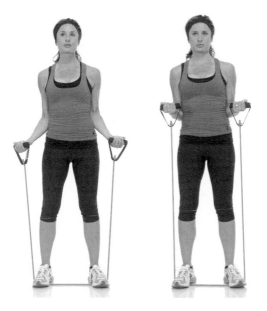

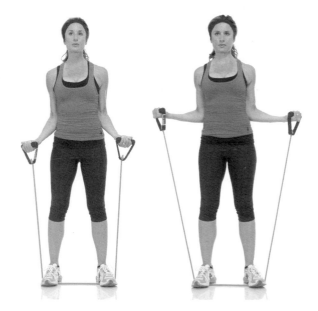

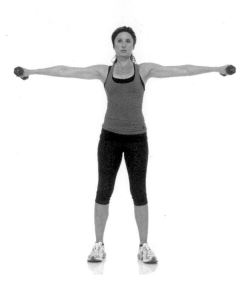

37. Shoulder Shapers

- *How to:* While holding a weight in each hand, stand with your feet hip-width apart, and your abs engaged. Lift your arms out to the sides until they're parallel with the floor. Raise your arms for a count of 5 seconds, hold for 2 seconds, then lower for 5 seconds. This move is designed to be super slow.

  - *Rock star muscle groups:* Shoulders

  - *Basic Tools:* Free weights

  - *Repetitions per set:* 15

  - *Level:* Gold

  - *Variation:* Try standing on one leg to work your stabilizing muscles.

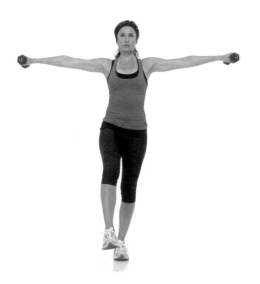

The Heart-Racer Power Moves

These are to be used as the In-between Exercise Pacer to keep your heart rate up. You may recognize some of these exercises from your elementary school days. Yes, remember, Rock Star Fitness is about going "back to basics."

They will be used as:

- Part of the circuit during the resistance training segment of the 14-Day Rock Star Boot Camp

- Exercises for your non cardio workout days—either as stand-alones or in combination—for a duration of no less than 20 minutes all together

Also, when for certain exercises I specify a time versus a number of reps, keep track of how many reps of an exercise you can do within a time frame so you can track your progress. It's about being the best you can be, so compete against yourself.

MIGHT AS WELL JUMP!

A lot of the Power Moves in this section involve jumping. Jump (also known as plyometric) training relies on explosive motion. Also, unlike traditional body sculpting workouts that focus on slow, controlled isolation exercises, plyometrics centers on full body movements that are great for toning all the major muscles in your body. Now I have switched them up in your 14-Day Rock Star Boot Camp, but as you continue and tweak the routine, remember to switch them up yourself. If you repeatedly exercise in the same way, your muscles switch to autopilot and the principle of diminishing returns applies. Basically, you won't see the same benefits.

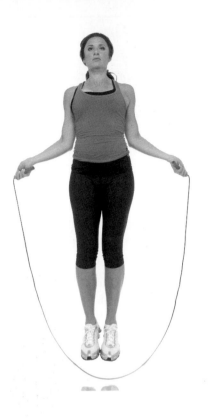

38. Jump Rope

- *How to:* Grab a skipping rope and start jumping like you did in grade school. Like riding a bike, though you may get rusty, you never forget this oldie but goodie.

  - *Rock Star muscle groups:* Calves, quads, abs/core, arms, heart

  - *Basic tool:* Skipping rope

  - *Repetitions per set:* 1 minute to start and work your way up to 3 minutes

  - *Level:* Gold; to make this Platinum, increase speed and duration; to make this Double Platinum, skip on one leg, alternating to the other leg after 1 minute

  - *Variation:* A weighted jump rope is a fantastic way to incorporate upper body work and increase the intensity 100 percent.

39. Straddle Jumps

- *How to:* Straddle step platform. Lower body into a semi-squat position. Jump up on to step using both legs. Keep the time from jumping down and up to a minimum. Feet should land softly on ground after each one.

  - *Rock star muscle groups:* Total lower body and heart

  - *Basic tool(s):* Step/platform

  - *Level:* Platinum

  - *Variation: Jumps on Step*
    1. Stand facing step platform with feet slightly wider than hip-width apart.
    2. Lower body into a semi-squat position and immediately jump up onto box. Do not hold a squat position before jumping up—keep the time between jumping down and jumping up to a minimum.
    3. Feet should land softly on step. Step back down (not jump back down if you're a beginner) and repeat.

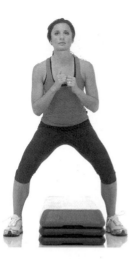

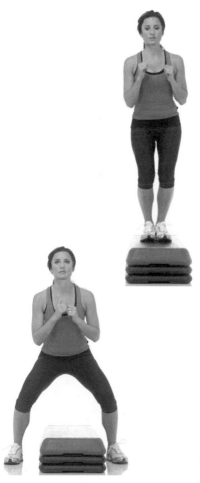

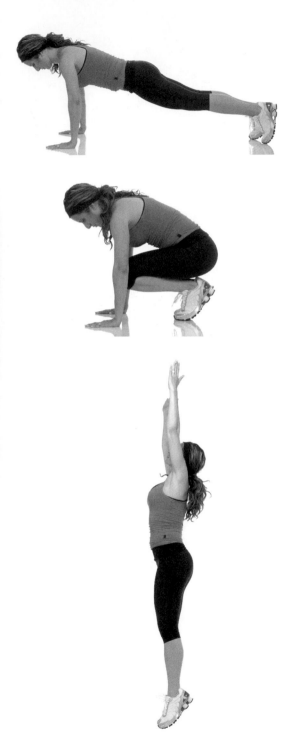

40. Burpee

- *How to:* Yet another exercise you likely did in elementary school. Assume a push-up position, then pull legs in toward your chest as you jump, raising your arms up in the air above your head.

  - *Rock Star muscle groups:* Abs/core, quads, hamstrings, shoulders

  - *Basic tool:* Just you

  - *Repetitions per set:* 12–15

  - *Level:* Gold

  - *Variation:* Add a medicine ball that you pick up and raise above your head with a jump up in the final stage, which makes this a Double Platinum exercise.

41. Mountain Climber

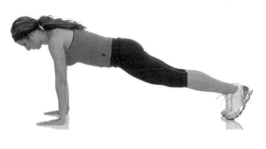

- *How to:* Start in a push-up position with your feet hip-width apart. Bend your knee and jump up, bringing your right thigh under the right side of your torso and leaving your left leg out behind you. Quickly jump your right leg back to starting position while simultaneously jumping your left knee in toward your torso. Please keep your pace as fast as possible and DON'T stick your glutes (butt) in the air.

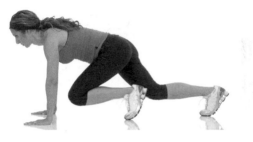

  - *Rock Star muscle groups:* Lower abs, transverse abs, chest, shoulders, legs, heart

  - *Basic tool:* Just you

  - *Repetitions per set:* 1 minute to start

  - *Level:* Platinum

  - *Variation:* Use a platform to place your hands on. This will make it Gold.

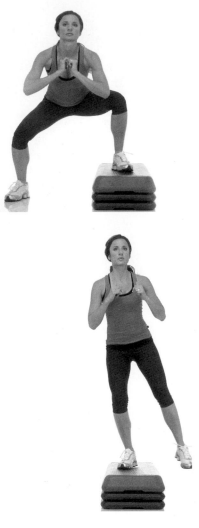

42. Lateral Power Lunge

- *How to:* Stand with your left foot on the floor next to a step or bench (or equivalent object). Push off the step or bench using your right leg and jump as high as possible. Reach forward and upwards for maximum height. Leap over the step or bench and land with your left foot on the step or bench and your right foot on the floor on the other side of the step, immediately bending your knees to absorb the impact. Repeat from this side.

- *Rock Star muscle groups:* Inner and outer thighs, glutes, quads, heart

- *Basic tool:* You

- *Repetitions per set:* Begin with 12 (1 rep is back and forth)

- *Level:* Gold/Platinum (holding light free weights makes this a Platinum exercise)

- *Variation:* Lateral Jumps (see below)

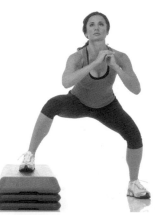

Those were my chart-topping five. Now here are some back-up performers that will make excellent stand-ins.

43. The Lateral Jump:

In this exercise, you will jump sideways back and forth over a line (you can lay your jump rope on the floor). Start on the right side of the line standing on the balls of your feet with your knees bent leaning forward slightly at the hips. Jump, pulling your knees up toward your chest and landing on the left side of the line. Keep going side to side for 30 seconds. Work your way up to 1 minute.

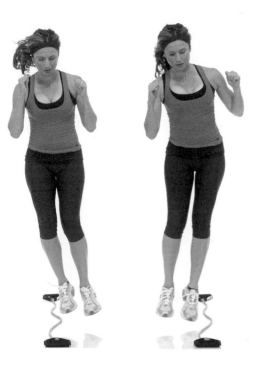

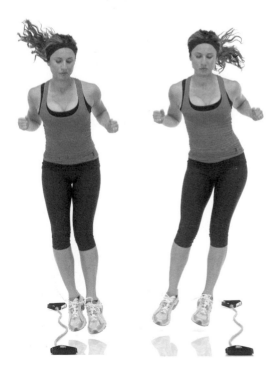

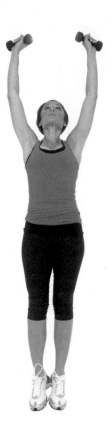

44. Jumping Jack

- *How to:* As with skipping, the jumping jack is an unforgettable throwback exercise from childhood. It's amazing how you can raise your heart rate quickly with this one. Make sure you fully extend your arms out over your head and that you land lightly (that is, no thumping like an elephant as you'll do damage to your knees over time).

- *Rock Star muscle groups:* Quads, calves, abs/core

- *Basic tool:* Just you

- *Repetitions per set:* 1 minute to start

- *Level:* Gold

- *Variation:* Holding a set of free weights makes this a Platinum-level exercise.

FORM AND FUNCTION

Even the most virtuoso of lead guitarists have been known to play the wrong power chord. Don't hit the wrong note while working out as it will throw everything off key. Here are my top 10 technique mistakes to avoid while exercising.

1. *Holding on while using the stair-master or any cardio machine:* Obtaining your balance and swinging your arms will promote calorie burning.

2. *The triceps swing:* Never bring your arms above 90 degrees while performing a triceps press-down either with a bar or rope.

3. *Holding your breath:* Make sure to exhale during the positive motion and inhale during the negative motion. For instance, exhale while standing up during a squat, and inhale on your way down.

4. *Dumbbell music:* Do not hit the dumbbells together during any exercise. By banging the dumbbells together, you lose control and the contraction of your muscles.

5. *Do not bounce while stretching:* Hold your position as bouncing can cause injury.

6. *Do not allow your knee to pass your toe while performing any exercise:* This is most common during the lunge. To avoid knee injuries, perform your exercises by keeping your knees steady at a 90-degree angle.

7. *The neck crunch:* Do not pull your neck when you crunch your abs. Let your head fall into your hands and focus on a spot with your eyes, if you lose that spot, you've pulled your neck too hard.

8. *The flapping wing curl:* There should be no space between your elbows and your body while performing a bicep curl.

9. *Heavy feet:* Float like a butterfly, sting like a bee. Try to be light on your feet. To avoid pounding your feet as a runner, try to glide rather than bounce.

10. *Dehydration:* The lack of water will decrease energy levels and fatigue leads to poor technique.

PART 3: 14-DAY ROCK STAR BOOT CAMP

Here is where we put it all together as your Part 1: Ultimate Cardio meets Part 2: Power Moves to move you closer to Rock Stardom on your own fit and healthy terms.

This 14-day Rock Star Boot Camp is designed to kick-start you to the next level of your fitness life. Follow the order of days as I present them. I have structured each circuit so that the next day's does not over-work any particular muscle group. Rest and recovery are as important to building muscle as is the actual workout. I have also factored in two rest days, one per week, for the very same reason. Fatigue is not fit. And remember to stick to your Ultimate Cardio program, which you will be performing concurrently for the best results.

If you haven't completed your Ultimate Cardio before you start your circuit, do your 5-minute warm-up first. And always finish with your cooldown and stretching.

Week 1

Day 1
- Jump rope, 2 minutes
- Walking lunges back and forth across a room (holding weights is optional)
- Standing side crunch, 12–15 reps
- Basic squat, 12–15 reps
- Push-ups, 10 reps
- Lying-down ball raises, 12–15
- Basic plank, 20–30 seconds
- Bicycle abs, 20 reps
- Basic plank, 20–30 sec
- Ball crunches, 20 reps
- Shoulder Shapers 12–15 reps (for intermediate and advanced, do them balancing on one leg to really activate your core; do half on one leg, then switch)

Repeat three times.

Day 2

- Mountain climber, 30 seconds; work up from there to 1 minute
- Plié squat, 15 reps
- Tricep dips, 12–15 reps (for the more advanced, one-handed tricep dips)
- Bulgarian lunges 12 reps each leg
- Bicep curls with resistance band 15 reps
- Leg lift in Swiss ball, 10 reps
- Leg curl with Swiss ball, 10 reps
- Alternating arm shoulder presses
- Plank, 30 seconds

Repeat three times

Day 3

- Speed Skating for 30 seconds
- Walk squat 21's
- Standing side crunch, 12–15 reps each side
- Stationary boxing jabs for 30 seconds
- Lying-down ball raises, 12–15 reps
- Basic Plank for 30 seconds,
- Bicycle abs, 25 reps
- Lying leg crossovers, "scissor sisters," 20 reps
- Lateral lunge with Shoulder raises 12–15 reps
- Stradle Jumps, 30 seconds (If you're a beginner do jumping jacks)
- Back extensions on ball, 12–15 reps

Repeat three times.

Day 4

- Burpees, 12–15 reps
- Single leg squats 12–15 reps (do a basic squat if you're a beginner)
- Chest press on ball, 12–15 reps
- Push-ups, 12 reps
- Crossover lunge with hammer curl, 12–15 reps

- Alternating arm shoulder press on ball, 10 reps
- Leg Curl with Swiss Ball, 12–15 reps
- Swiss ball leg pull in 10–12 reps
- Lying-down ball raises, 12–15 reps
- Side-lying triangle with ball each side, 12–15 reps each side (do without ball if you're a beginner)
- Plank 30 sec
- Ball Crunch 20 reps

Repeat three times.

Day 5

- Jump rope, 2 minutes
- Walking lunge with twist, back and forth across the room
- Shoulder Shapers, 12–15 reps
- Lateral lunges, 12–15 reps (do this with or without step and with or without shoulder raise)
- Back extension on ball, 12–15 reps
- Swiss ball leg pull in, set of 12–15/ ball crunches if this is to difficult
- Ball or Basic Plank, 30 seconds
- Lying-down ball raises, 12–15 reps
- Lying leg crossovers, "scissor sisters," 20 reps
- Mountain Climbers 30 sec
- Plié squats with overhead tricep extension, 15 reps
- Tricep dips, 12–15 reps

Repeat three times.

Day 6

- Jump rope, 2 minutes
- Lunge 10:1 hut and reverse (only go up to 6:1 if you're a beginner and work your way up)
- Side crunches, 12–15 each side
- Stationary boxing jabs 30 seconds
- Jumping Jack squats (holding light weight optional), 15 reps

- Walkover push-ups, 10 reps (do a set of regular push ups if this is too difficult)
- Bicycle crunches, 25 reps
- Reverse crunches, 12–15 reps
- Ball Plank, 30 seconds
- Crab walk, one side of the room and back.

Repeat 3 times

Day 7: Rest

Week 2

Day 8

- Speed skate, 1 minute
- Stationary boxing jabs, 30 seconds
- Reverse lunges 12–15 reps
- One handed Tricep Dips with one leg out 8–10 reps each side
- Lateral lunge with shoulder raise, 12–15 reps
- Plié squats, 20 reps
- Lateral jumps, 30 seconds
- Push-up with exercise ball, 12–15 reps
- Basic plank, 30 seconds; if you can after the 30 seconds, don't drop but instead pull alternate knee in to the opposite side; do this for 15 reps (this is a plank twist)
- Lying-down ball raises, 12–15 reps
- Lying leg crossovers, "scissor sisters," 20 reps
- Shoulder Shapers, 12–15 reps

Repeat three times.

Day 9

- Mountain climber, 1 minute
- Side crunches, 15 reps per side
- Reverse lunges, 15–20 (if you're more advanced, try doing this while holding a weighted medicine ball in front of you; fully extend your arms at shoulder height)
- Alternating shoulder arm press, 10 reps, 8 reps and so on
- Chest press on ball and crunch, 12–15 reps
- Back extension on ball, 12–15 reps
- Ball Crunch 20 reps
- Swiss ball leg pull-in, 12–15 reps
- Swiss Ball leg curl 12–15 (try doing single leg curls for 10 reps)

Repeat three times.

Day 10

- Speed skating, 1 minute
- Tricep dips, 15 reps
- Bicep curls with resistant band
- *Lunge 10 Hut (10:1)
- Shoulder Shapers 12–15 reps
- Straddle jumps, 30 seconds (do jumping jacks or lateral jumps if this is too difficult)
- Lying leg raises, 15 reps
- Plank for 30 seconds and then plank with twist, for 20 reps

Repeat three times.

Note: Since lunges are so effective, you will be sore the next day. I usually try to have a more extensive upper-body workout the following day because my legs are wiped, hence Day 11.

Day 11

- Jump rope, 2 minutes
- Walkover push-ups (alternative Swiss ball push-ups), 12–15 reps
- Alternating arm and shoulder presses, 12–15 reps]
- Chest press on ball, 12–15 reps
- Swing kicks, 20 reps
- Side lying triangle with or (without ball), 15 reps each side
- Back extensions on Swiss ball, 12–15 reps
- Stationary boxing jabs, 30 seconds
- Crab walk, back and forth from one side of the room and back

Repeat three times.

Day 12

- Jumping Jacks with light free weights, 1 minute
- Bulgarian lunges, 12–15 reps each side
- One-handed tricep dips with 1-leg out 8–10 reps each side
- Plank with alternating leg outs, 30 seconds
- Side-lying triangle with or without ball, 12–15 reps both sides
- Lying-down leg raises, 12–15 reps
- Lying leg crossovers, "scissor sisters", 20 reps
- Ball Crunch, 20 reps
- Ball Plank, 30 seconds
- One leg squat, 10 reps each side

Repeat three times.

Day 13

- Lateral power lunge, 1 minute
- Shoulder Shapers 12–15 reps
- Crossover lunge with hammer curl, 12–15 reps
- Boxing jabs, 30 seconds
- Plié squat, 20 reps
- Alternating shoulder arm raises, 10 reps
- Crunch on ball, 25 reps

- Reverse lunges 15 reps
- Bicep curls with resistant band

Repeat three times.

DON'T STOP BELIEVING

Congratulations! You have completed the 14-Day Rock Star Fitness Boot Camp. After this two-week period you may want to give it an encore, and go through the cycle again. Or you can slightly dial back to my recommended regular schedule, which will still promote weight loss. Do your circuit workout four times a week and your interval training cardio five or six days a week. To avoid falling into that dreaded workout rut, design your own circuits by mixing and matching the Power Moves to your heart's content. The possibilities are endless and the results will be unbelievable. But you believe it, so you will achieve it.

CHAPTER 5

ROCK STAR

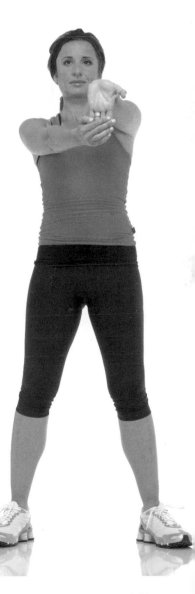

SO THIS IS IT. JUST LIKE A BUTTERFLY
emerging from its cocoon or Kelly Clarkson winning on "American
Idol," you are ready to step out into the lights and be the Rock Star of
your life. You know so much more now. You know that your body is
beautiful; you know how to motivate yourself; you know what to eat
and what not to eat; and you know the best way to work out for the best
results. You also feel so much better than you did before. And because
of this, you know that your life will never be the same again.

Life is made up of the everyday, and I bet you are determined to get
through each one without getting any dust on your shine. You want to
keep working it the Rock Star Fitness way, and I understand that. But
you don't have to "perfect" nine to five, 24/7, seven days a week. That's
just too much pressure, just like those Hollywood standards that are
impossible to maintain.

Remember that Rock Star Fitness is realistic and designed to be
easily integrated into your life, so keep it real. You won't do all the
dos in this book and you'll definitely do some of the don'ts. Even I still
have artificial sweetener in my life sometimes. It's not the best choice,
but we're all human, right? I still use my cheat day as well—for fries
and pizza.

I know that you will really want to maintain the principles and follow the guidelines, but I trust that you'll do what you gotta do to make
it work for you. I have a friend who just can't give up her 250-calorie

latte twice a day in favor of a healing tea, but she switched from grande to tall, and has shaved off some of those calories. It's about making better choices. You can do all our Rock Star mental motivation exercises, or you can buy a cute outfit a size or two smaller, then set a target date for when you will fit into it. That's fine if that is what it takes for you to crank that treadmill sky high.

In this chapter I will address The Day in the Life of You, the Rock Star. From the things you shouldn't live without to Rock Star work sheets, I am striking the show in a way that will help keep you going now that the tour is over.

First, I will share the choices I make on a typical day. Get ready for my "Jenniferisms"—my own little habits—that some may consider quirky and may be against the conventional wisdom. For instance, a lot of people recommend eating a wide variety foods to avoid boredom. The Jenniferism is that I try to eat the same thing or very similar things every day. Or at the very least I have one routine meal as it establishes consistency. You don't even think about experimenting and thus are in a better position to avoid pitfalls.

My wish is that my choices will inspire you to create and develop your own Rock Star make-it-work-for-you habits.

A DAY IN THE LIFE

Between 7 a.m. and 7:30 a.m.: I wake up and have breakfast to kickstart my metabolism into a burning state. I like to eat clean protein. It could be five egg whites with a bit of low-fat cheese, or yogurt and berries. Sometimes I'll have a Whey Protein Powder Shake, which will have a bit of fruit and ice, which is a great source of clean, high-quality protein.

Between 8 a.m. and 9 a.m: I work out whenever I can and, in another Jenniferism, I have my one cup of coffee with a drop of low fat milk and Splenda or stevia just before to really kick things off. I like working out in the morning because it gets the day off to a good start psychologically. You feel like you have accomplished something and you will be more cognizant of what you eat the rest of the day. Also, your endorphins kick in, so you start your day off happy! By the way, each of your workouts should take about 20–30 minutes depending on your fitness level. That doesn't include your cardio, of course!

After my workout, I start with my work day, which includes working with personal clients, meetings, and other business ventures I am involved in. If I have a very early morning meeting or client and am not able to work out in the morning, I will try and use my lunch hour for my workout since the later it gets, the more chance there is that I won't do it. I make a point of scheduling it in my day timer (Blackberry) like I would any other meeting.

Lunch: If I am going to work out during my lunch hour, I will eat an apple just prior for that natural burst of energy. As I noted earlier, research shows you can work out 10 minutes longer after eating an apple.

If I've worked out in the morning, I eat a clean, lean protein like turkey, with a complex carb right after as I need to keep fueled up! If I've worked out at mid-day at a round 2 p.m., I'll have a huge salad with a lean protein

Mid-afternoon: I snack on another apple. In yet another Jenniferism, I will drink half a Diet Coke (I know, I know) or Hanson Diet Soda, which has Splenda in it instead of aspartame.

Dinner: I have a big, big, big green salad with a clean protein.

I try and eat at least two hours before bedtime, so my body has a bit of time to digest. Eating too close to bedtime can disrupt sleep. Also, to stave off late-night cravings, I brush my teeth right after dinner. My mouth gets that pristine feeling and my mind gets the signal that I'm done.

Tip: Rinse your mouth with mouthwash or brush your teeth when you feel that emotional hunger come on (when your bored and just think your hungry). It minimizes the craving to eat after and breaks the cycle of your obsessive thought.

All through the day I drink water in some form, usually herbal teas and green tea in the winter months. This helps give me the feeling of being full.

Also, in another Jenniferism, I chew gum (A LOT)—Orbit Sugar-

Free Bubble Mint—to satiate my out-of-control oral fixation. I also sometimes have a Sorbee Suckers moment—each has Splenda in it too, also both satisfy that sugar craving.

Tip: Sucking frozen fruit when you have a sweet craving does the trick also. My favorite is Mango and grapes. Both take a while to eat so it slows me down from having a pound of it and it's a great substitute for eating candy.

That was a typical day in my life, and you will have your typical days too, but we both know that not every day will be typical. Sometimes, and quite often, I'm sure, you'll go out to eat. What happens is what I like to call Saturday Night Sabotage. You know, when you have been doing just fine on your eating plan, and then you decide to go out to dinner with a friend. It starts with a responsible glass of red wine—after all it's only 150 calories and good for your heart. But then the defenses go down and you're eating all that refined flour in the bread basket. And after a couple more glasses, creamy pasta and dessert seem like a fabulous idea! But even if you stay mindful and it's a Wednesday lunch with a colleague, there is sabotage lurking in that menu.

Here's how to offset it:

1. Even if you exercise iron self-control, restaurants are where boundaries fall away. Think about what you are doing and chew slowly as the brain takes about 20 minutes to register that you're full. Have a bottle of water on the table. Drink a lot of it, especially if you feel a craving coming on. Half the time, what you think is hunger is actually dehydration.

2. Lay off the liquor. It has nothing but empty calories that turn straight into sugar and causes you to eat way more than you normally would. Order a cranberry and soda (with a higher proportion of soda) with a twist of lime. At least soda looks like vodka!

3. Unless it's nouvelle cuisine, restaurant main course portions tend to be outlandishly large. Order two appetizers instead and make

sure one is a green salad with a vinaigrette dressing.

4. Even if you order "clean," because of oil transfer that happens in any busy kitchen, or seasonings and dressings you did not realize were part of the dish, factor in at least 300 more stealth calories.

5. Avoid anything that is sautéed, breaded, battered, coated, and pan-fried. These mouth-watering words translate to fat, fat, fat on a plate. Instead, opt for dishes that are grilled, steamed, baked, broiled, or poached.

6. Celebrities do it all the time, and the most reputable, service-oriented establishments treat all their customers like one. Ask for variations on your meal if you see no healthy options. If ever there was a time to unleash your inner Rock Star, this is it.

And that's just going out for a formal dining experience, but as you run around just living your life—noshing while shopping or grabbing an extra smoothie for the road trip or hanging out and someone orders Chinese—you may take a time out from the Rock Star principles. Consider it your cheat day by accident and just use it to replace your intended cheat day. It turns out that 1 pound of fat is 3,500 calories, so it takes just 500 extra calories a day that are not burned off for you to gain a pound a week. I have created some hypothetical situations that are all too common to remind you how quickly those 500 calories can accumulate. This calorie count will break it all down for you and help you be mindful of your math.

MONDAY MOVIE NIGHT
1 small Diet Coke (0 calories) + 1 small bag of buttered popcorn (400 calories) + 1 box of raisonetttes (190 calories) = 590 calories

TUESDAY TAKEOUT WITH BOYFRIEND AND BEST FRIEND
1 Chinese beer + General Tso chicken (437 calories) + broccoli in black bean sauce (57 calories) + steamed white rice (90 calories) + 1 fortune cookie (35 calories) = 619 calories

WEDNESDAY MID-AFTERNOON STARBUCKS RUN

1 grande skim milk latte with chocolate sprinkles (135 calories) + Starbucks Crispy marshmallow square (360 calories) + 1 Starbucks mini chocolate chip cookie (120 calories) = 615 calories

THURSDAY NIGHT DRINKS WITH THE GIRLS

2 flutes of champagne (182 calories) + half a bowl of bar nuts (200 calories) + 3 caviar blinis (162 calories) = 544 calories

FRIDAY ALL-MORNING BOARDROOM BRAINSTORM

1 black coffee with Splenda (5 calories) + 1 glass of grapefruit juice (96 calories) + 1 handful of red grapes (30 calories) + 1 butter croissant (340 calories) + 1 bran muffin (190 calories) + 2 orange wedges (16 calories) = 677 calories

SATURDAY SHOPPING

1 skim milk latte + 1 glass of orange juice + scrambled eggs with toast at brunch (500 calories) + 1 slice of pizza and a Diet Coke (272 calories) + fries (100 calories) = 872 calories

SUNDAY AFTERNOON HIGH TEA

2 cups of Earl Grey with milk and sugar (36 calories) + 4 ham finger sandwiches (255 calories) + 1 slice of apple pie with a scoop of vanilla ice cream (324 calories) = 615 calories

Eating 500 rogue calories is not the end of the world—I've built cheat days into Rock Star Fitness anyway—especially if you get right back on the wagon and keep on staying with the Rock Star food principles. Also, cheat day or no cheat day, your working out must remain consistent— the cheat day is allowed only if you burn those extra calories off. Just to refresh your memory, four days of resistance training and five days of cardio are supposed to be constants in your life. Speaking of constants, there are a few other things that are just non-negotiable.

I CANT LIVE IF LIVING IS WITHOUT....

Water: We all know how important water is and that we should drink at least eight glasses of it a day, but how many of you still don't? Simply put, you cannot underestimate the infinite benefits of drinking half a gallon to 1 gallon of water a day, and remember, distilled water is best because it's sodium-free. Check the labels for salt.

Water is basically the alpha and the omega. It helps organs function, absorbs all essential vitamins and minerals, regulates body temperature, helps your stomach to produce digestive enzymes, and is a natural detoxifier as it helps to flush the system. Start drinking all the water you are supposed to and I guarantee that your skin will be much clearer and your eyes brighter and whiter.

If you don't get enough water, you will become dehydrated. You can tell your dehydration level by the color of your urine. If it's dark yellow rather than light, you are dehydrated. Dehydration can lead to fatigue, lethargy, headaches, blurred vision, irritability, constipation, and high cholesterol. And if vanity is your key motivator, thirst is often mistaken for hunger, hence overeating. Dehydration has also been linked to weight gain and cellulite. Ironically, dehydration also causes fluid retention—that's bloating to you—as the body goes into starvation mode and hangs onto any water just in case it does not get anymore. Drink up.

Multivitamins: If we were all eating well and our soil nutrient quality hadn't degraded as much as it has over the last few decades, we wouldn't even need to consider taking multivitamins. With the right combination of high-nutrient foods, all vitamin needs should be covered, but that doesn't always happen.

No multivitamin (or supplement, for that matter) is a substitute for a good diet, but take a multivitamin to fill in any gaps. Look for store name/white-label brands as they are usually less expensive and of high quality.

Your multivitamin should have at least 100 percent of the daily requirements of vitamins A, C, D, E, K, B1, B2, B6, B12, and folic acid. It should have at least 50 percent of iodine, copper, zinc, and selenium. Also, women should bear in mind that we need more iron than men because of the menstrual cycle, and your multivitamin should have approximately 18 milligrams of iron in it. But note that more isn't necessarily better with vitamin dosages, especially when it comes to fat-soluble vitamins such as vitamins A and D, which become toxic when taken at high levels.

Those who exercise regularly and vigorously—and that means all you Rock Stars—should also be taking a calcium-magnesium supplement. These help the body deal with and respond to the stress of weight lifting and vigorous exercise. Note that a calcium-magnesium supplement must have vitamin D in it as well as it's needed to absorb the calcium. Speaking of absorption, multivitamins should always be taken with a meal as they are absorbed better with food and can upset an empty stomach. Also, never take your vitamin with coffee since caffeine inhibits the absorption.

Coenzyme Q10: Your cells use coenzymes to produce the energy your body needs for cell growth and maintenance. Coenzyme Q10 works to digest food and perform other body processes, and helps protect the heart and skeletal muscles. It is also an antioxidant. The body makes its own CoQ10 as part of the normal metabolic process, but as we age, we make considerably less, so we need to get it else-where. CoQ10 is naturally present in small amounts in a wide variety of foods, but levels are particularly high in organ meats such as heart, liver, and kidney, as well as beef, soy oil, sardines, mackerel, and peanuts. If you choose to use this, follow the label directions unless you have a nutritional consultation with a nutritionist, dietitian, or doctor.

And don't stop there. Always make a point of:

1. *Going outside:* Get out of the office and walk around the block a couple of times a day. Sunlight is a natural source of vitamin D. It also triggers the release of serotonin, which is a mood lifter and lowers stress.

2. *Sitting down:* Research shows that those who eat while standing up, and we've all been guilty of that, consume about 184 more calories a meal than those who sat down and ate from a plate.

3. *Being prepared:* Stash healthy food options such as natural (raw) nuts, oatmeal, and trail mix at your desk or in your car so you won't be forced to make a bad choice.

4. *Seeing your friends:* People who are lonely have more stress-related problems.

5. *Don't drink too much:* More than one alcoholic drink a day can raise your risk of breast cancer.

6. *Getting enough sleep:* Sleep deprivation has been linked to weight gain as it decreases the human growth hormone that regulates the body's ratio of fat and muscle. It also triggers cortisol, that lovely substance linked to belly fat. Sleeplessness also causes depression.

7. *Have sex first:* Apart from the calorie-burning, metabolism-boosting benefits, women who have sex at least once a week have better immune function.

And we cannot speak about a day in the life without talking about beauty. For better or for worse, we spend lots of time, morning and night, looking at the woman in the mirror and slathering on expensive creams that claim to tighten skin, take out wrinkles, and essentially perform plastic surgery in a jar! Cosmetic companies are not allowed to guarantee results. These creams do feel nice, smell nice, and do improve the appearance of skin, but they function only topically and temporarily. To take real preventative measures and turn back the clock, open your fridge, not your bathroom cabinet. The old adage that beauty starts from the inside out has never been truer than in this case, and the skin is a great indicator of what is going on in the body: good skin means good health.

We have already counted the ways in which water will make you gorgeous. It will also plump up your skin and reduce fine lines, and it only costs about $2 for a really big bottle. Crème de la Mer costs about $200 for a really, really small bottle. Nuff said. Just eat instead, and when you do, eat these:

Apples: You know by now that they are at the top of all my lists, but this magic fruit also has properties that can help relieve eczema and cleanse the system by detoxifying the liver.

Blueberries: Good things come in small packages as the tiny blueberries have 40 percent more antioxidant capacity than strawberries. They are high in vitamin C, which promotes collagen formation—important to keep the skin from sagging. They also enhance circulation—good news for the skin. So go blue and go organic to avoid the pesticides.

Fish oils: The essential fatty acids in fish oils encourage the production of strong collagen and elastin fibers, which fight sagging and keep the skin hydrated. Bye-bye fine lines and wrinkling. They also have an anti-inflammatory effect on the skin, which is strong enough to fight eczema and chronic skin conditions. They also prevent hair loss. To get your EFAs, eat wild salmon and wild tuna. I highly recommend supplementing with a distilled fish oil supplement daily. Make sure it is from a reputable company like Genuine Health. Select one that has been distilled (to remove artificial chemicals), is enteric-coated (so it is easy on your intestines), and is made with wild or smaller fish such as anchovies and sardines. The shorter lifespan of smaller fish means that they have had less exposure to toxins.

Tomatoes: They are a fantastic antiwrinkle treatment as they are rich in the powerful plant chemical called lycopene, which has been shown to reduce skin cell damage and redness. Lycopene is also known for its blood-purifying and natural detoxification qualities. In order to best absorb lycopene, it needs to be mixed with a healthy fat. Drizzle some extra-virgin olive oil over your fresh tomatoes, which should be organic.

Sunflower seeds: Rich in vitamins, protein, and minerals, these tasty treats provide all the skin's essential nutrients. They are an excellent source of the fat-soluble vitamin E, shown to prevent damage from free radicals, which cause the cellular-level aging that shows up as wrinkles. Sprinkle them over a salad or munch on a handful as a solo snack.

I know that you will enjoy the benefits of all these beauty boosters, but come to think of it, No Gym Required is a beauty booster in and of itself. Accepting yourself is beautiful, committing to yourself is beautiful, being healthy and in shape is beautiful. You are beautiful and will only get better and better as you continue in all your Rock Star glory. I leave you with the Rock Star personal trainer work sheets. They will help you to keep all the key information in one place and follow what is sure to be your absolutely amazing progress. Please let me know how your tour is going at IROCK@nogymrequired.com. And while you're at it, believe it. Achieve it. Rock on.

CHAPTER 6

THE NO GYM REQUIRED MENU PLAN

NOTE FOR VEGETARIANS

It is easy to substitute tofu in many of the chicken or meat recipes. You can also try using tempeh (a type of soy) for a nutty, protein-rich option. It is important as a vegetarian to get enough protein to manage carb cravings and build lean muscle. If you are tired, you may want to ensure you are getting enough iron and B12 because both are hard to get on a veggie diet and are critical nutrients for energy production. Great vegetarian iron sources include the following:

		Amount of Iron
Lentils, cooked	1 cup	6.6 milligrams
Spinach, cooked	1 cup	6.4 milligrams
Quinoa, cooked	1 cup	6.3 milligrams
Tofu	4 ounces	6.0 milligrams
Tempeh	1 cup	4.8 milligrams
Lima beans, cooked	1 cup	4.4 milligrams
Swiss chard, cooked	1 cup	4.0 milligrams

It is harder to get vitamin B12, which is available only in meat, milk products, and eggs, so if you are a vegan, it is important to consider taking a supplement.

Tip: A cup of snap peas contain only 30 calories and 4 grams of fiber. That is twice as much an average piece of whole-grain bread or bowl of cereal! Like protein and healthy fats, fiber does a great job of slowing down sugars so they won't hit you all at once.

1 cup raw snap peas
1 serving:
Calories: 30
Fat: 0 grams
Carbs: 8 grams (4 of which are fiber)
Protein: 4 grams

WEEK 1

MEAL	Day 1	Day 2	Day 3
Breakfast 400 Calories	Scrambled Egg Whites Goat Cheese Whole Grain Toast Orange	Prepared Oatmeal Mixed Berries Greek Yogurt	*Chocolate Banana Protein Shake*
Snack 150 Calories	Wasa Cracker Smoked Salmon Fat Free Cream Cheese	Instant Miso Soup Celery Peanut Butter or Almond Butter	Shelled Edamame
Lunch 400 Calories	*Mix and Match Salad* *Voila Vinaigrette* Whole Grain Roll	*Mix and Match Salad* *Voila Vinaigrette* Whole Grain Roll	*Mix and Match Salad* *Voila Vinaigrette* Whole Grain Roll
Snack 150 Calories	Carrot Sticks Sunflower Seeds	Air Popped Popcorn Parmesan Cheese Green Pumpkin Seeds	*Easy Yogurt Dip* Sliced Jicama Carrot Sticks
Dinner 400 Calories	Lean Steak Baked Sweet Potato Steamed Broccoli	*Quinoa & Veggie Bowl* Natural Almonds	Grilled Chicken Breast Brown Rice Steamed Asparagus Sliced Tomato Balsamic Vinegar
Note: Italic type in menu designates recipes.			

Day 4	Day 5	Day 6	Day 7
Skinny Breakfast Sandwich Orange	Kashi GoLean Cereal Skim Milk Strawberries	*Mediterranean Egg White Omelet* Whole Grain Toast Grapefruit Honey	*Apple Cinnamon Amaranth* Greek yogurt
Kiwi Green Pumpkin Seeds	*Hollywood Hummus* Red Pepper	Apple Part-Skim String Cheese	*Hollywood Hummus* Red Pepper
Mix and Match Salad *Voila Vinaigrette* Whole Grain Roll	*Mix and Match Salad* *Voila Vinaigrette* Whole Grain Roll	*Mix and Match Salad* *Voila Vinaigrette* Whole Grain Roll	*Mix and Match Salad* *Voila Vinaigrette* Whole Grain Roll
Cottage Cheese Cantaloupe	Sliced Roasted Turkey Breast Lettuce Havarti Cheese	Wasa Cracker Almond Butter Strawberries	Air Popped Popcorn Parmesan Cheese Green Pumpkin Seeds
White Fish *Spicy Sweet Potato Wedges* Steamed Peas	*Good Times Gazpacho* Avocado Cooked Shrimp Wasa Crackers	Grilled Tofu *Voila Vinaigrette* Brown Rice Steamed Baby Bok Choy	*Herbed Salmon Packets* Mashed Cauli-flower Steamed Peas

TOTAL = 1500 CALORIES PER DAY

WEEK 2

MEAL	Day 8	Day 9	Day 10
Breakfast **400 Calories**	Hard Boiled Eggs Whole Grain Toast Banana	Kashi GoLean Cereal Skim Milk Strawberries	*Apple Cinnamon* *Amaranth* Greek yogurt
Snack **150 Calories**	Apple Part-Skim String Cheese	Shelled Edamame	*Easy Yogurt Dip* Sliced Jicama Carrot Sticks
Lunch **400 Calories**	*Mix and Match* *Salad* *Voila Vinaigrette* Whole Grain Roll	*Mix and Match* *Salad* *Voila Vinaigrette* Whole Grain Roll	*Mix and Match* *Salad* *Voila Vinaigrette* Whole Grain Roll
Snack **150 Calories**	*Hollywood* *Hummus* Carrot Sticks	Celery Peanut Butter or Almond Butter	Kiwi Green Pumpkin Seeds
Dinner **400 Calories**	Grilled Chicken Breast *Spicy Sweet Potato* *Wedges* Steamed Asparagus Cherry Tomatoes	Solid Gold Soup Whole Grain Toast Swiss Cheese	White Fish Roasted Baby Potatoes Roasted Parsnips *Voila Vinaigrette*
Note: Italic type in menu designates recipes.			

Day 11	Day 12	Day 13	Day 14
Skinny Breakfast Sandwich Orange	*Chocolate Banana Protein Shake*	*Mediterranean Egg White Omelet* Whole Grain Toast Grapefruit Honey	Prepared Oatmeal Mixed Berries Greek Yogurt
Apple Sunflower Seeds	*Easy Yogurt Dip* Sliced Jicama Carrot Sticks	Sunflower Seeds Carrot Sticks	Wasa Cracker Smoked Salmon Fat Free Cream Cheese
Mix and Match Salad *Voila Vinaigrette* Whole Grain Roll	*Mix and Match Salad* *Voila Vinaigrette* Whole Grain Roll	*Mix and Match Salad* *Voila Vinaigrette* Whole Grain Roll	*Mix and Match Salad* *Voila Vinaigrette* Whole Grain Roll
Hollywood Hummus Red Pepper	Air Popped Popcorn Parmesan Cheese Green Pumpkin Seeds	Sliced Roasted Turkey Breast Lettuce Havarti Cheese	Pineapple Chunks Walnut Halves
Balsamic Salmon Ribbons Steamed Greens Broccoli Brown Rice	Instant Miso Soup *Asian Chicken Lettuce Wraps* Avocado Tomato	*Quinoa & Veggie Bowl* Natural Almonds	Shrimp and Edamame Stir-Fry Brown Rice
TOTAL = 1500 CALORIES PER DAY			

THE TWO WEEK PLAN

This two-week meal plan makes it easy for you to start eating meals that provide the best fuel for your body while still controlling calories and fat. Based on the advice provided in Chapter 3, following this plan will help you to establish better eating habits, making a nutritious diet something you can follow long term. A couple of key points to remember:

1. When shopping for this meal plan, whenever possible, buy local and choose organic vegetables, fruit, breads, and dairy products.

2. Each day's menu contains about 1500 calories; this amount of energy will promote weight loss for a moderately active person. If you plan on being exceptionally active, add an extra snack to ensure that you have enough energy to fuel your activities. (It is important to balance caloric intake with your activity level in order to make weight loss both safe and sustainable.)

3. Each menu contains the same number of calories for each meal and snack; breakfast, lunch, and dinner are each about 400 calories and each snack is about 150 calories. This makes the snacks and meals interchangeable throughout the week. If there is a menu suggestion that you don't love, simply substitute one from another day that you do! By learning how these portions add up, using this menu plan will help you to choose the appropriate portions of food when creating your own meals.

4. Including protein rich foods and complex carbohydrates throughout the day is key to feeling satisfied and to avoid the urge to binge between meals. For vegetarians, substitute tofu, tempeh, or other sources of complete proteins for the meat options provided.

5. It is important to drink plenty of fluids (such as water and tea) with meals and throughout the day to keep hydrated and to curb cravings. Caffeinated teas such as white or green tea are an antioxidant rich alternative for your morning coffee. Drinking a hot beverage such as tea or even hot water whenever you have a

hunger craving can hydrate and curb snacking at the same time. And, for an energy charging pick-me-up, steep ginseng tea for your afternoon snack.

6. Have a kitchen scale and measuring cups on hand for this first two-week period to ensure that you are eating the portion sizes used to calculate the calorie counts. Portion distortion is a huge contributor to unconscious overeating.

7. Don't skip the snacks! The combination of complex carb-rich fruits and vegetables with a protein source will prevent hunger pangs throughout the day. Be sure to use unsalted nuts and seeds to control sodium.

8. Eating a big salad everyday is an easy way to include plenty of antioxidant-rich veggies in your diet and you'll feel like you are having a satisfying meal. To keep things simple, the meal plan calls for salads at lunch but they can be eaten as a dinner option as well.

9. All the recipes are designed to serve two people. However, the recipes double easily to serve four.

10. This menu doesn't include desserts although there is plenty of fresh fruit to satisfy your sweet tooth. If you are still craving a sweet snack, have a few low calorie desserts (50 calories or less) such as sugarfree Fudgesicles or puddings on hand to have as an indulgence once and a while. As long as you limit yourself to a couple of treats a week, it will help you keep on track without compromising your goals.

DAY 1

Let's get started! The key to today's menu is to remember to prepare foods with little or no added fat or sugar. Most plain rolled oats have easy on-package preparation instructions to make a hot cereal; they're a better option than the instant sweetened versions. Today's lunch recipe is the *Mix-and-Match 'Big' Salad,* which will become a daily staple.

Breakfast
6 scrambled egg whites
1/4 cup crumbled goat cheese or shredded Cheddar cheese
1 piece whole grain toast
1 orange

Snack
1 Wasa cracker
2 pieces smoked salmon or lox
2 tbsp fat free cream cheese

Lunch
1 portion **Mix-and-Match 'Big' Salad (pg 159)**
1 whole grain roll

Snack
3 tbsp toasted sunflower seeds
1/2 cup carrot sticks

Dinner
4 oz grilled or broiled lean steak (loin, tenderloin, or round cuts)
1 small (4 oz) baked sweet potato
1 cup steamed broccoli

Daily Total: 1500 calories

Mix-and-Match 'Big' Salad

Using the following suggestions as inspiration, you can have a different salad for each menu day. The greens and vegetables are interchangeable, however, to control calories choose only two portions from the protein section.

4 cups leafy greens such as
- Belgian endive
- Boston lettuce
- red or green leaf lettuce
- romaine lettuce
- iceberg lettuce
- mixed fresh herbs
- spinach
- arugula
- watercress

2 cups mixed assorted vegetables such as
- shredded red, green or napa cabbage
- diced cooked beets
- broccoli florets
- sliced carrots

- chopped tomatoes
- sliced sweet peppers
- sliced cucumber
- sliced mushrooms
- sliced celery
- blanched asparagus spears
- fresh shelled garden peas
- blanched green beans
- cooked corn
- chopped cooked sweet potatoes
- sliced red or green onion
- sprouts

Any 2 portions of the following protein sources:
- 1 cup chopped, cooked, boneless, skinless, free-range chicken breast

- 4 oz cooked wild salmon, flaked
- 5 oz drained canned wild tuna, packed in water
- 3 oz sliced, grilled grain-fed lean steak (such as round or loin cuts)
- 5 oz peeled, cooked white shrimp
- 3/4 cup cubed, cooked tofu
- 3/4 cups frozen, shelled edamame
- 2/3 cups cooked lentils
- 2/3 cups cooked chick peas
- 3/4 cups cooked black beans
- 2 hard boiled eggs
- 3 tbsp toasted walnuts
- 5 tbsp toasted almonds
- 3 tbsp toasted sunflower seeds
- 3 tbsp flax seed
- 2 tbsp Voila Vinaigrette (pg 161)

Toss all ingredients in a big bowl until combined. Makes 2 servings.

Nutrients per serving: 316 calories, 14 g fat, 13 g carbohydrates, 6 g fiber, 36 g protein, 296 mg sodium. Excellent source of vitamin A, vitamin C, folate, niacin, and magnesium.

[Note: Nutritional analysis is based on a composite salad using a variety of the suggested ingredients.]

Tip: You can substitute your own favorite gourmet salad dressing for the *Voila Vinaigrette.* Rather than creamy dressings that can be high in fat and sodium, read the labels and choose vinaigrette-style dressings that contain wholesome ingredients such canola or olive oil.

DAY 2

When preparing today's breakfast, cook a couple of extra eggs to use as a salad topper later in the week. Place a page marker on the vinaigrette recipe, you'll be using it everyday in your lunchtime salad and it makes a great finishing glaze for your cooked chicken, beef, fish, or tofu.

Breakfast
 1 cup prepared oatmeal
 1 cup mixed berries
 1 1/4 cup plain Greek-style or probiotic yogurt

Snack
 1 cup instant miso soup
 1 celery stalk
 1 tbsp natural peanut butter or almond butter

Lunch
 1 portion *Mix-and-Match 'Big' Salad (pg 159)*
 1 whole grain roll

Snack
 2 cups plain air popped popcorn
 1 tbsp grated Parmesan cheese
 1 tbsp toasted green pumpkin seeds

Dinner
 1 portion *Quinoa and Veggie Bowl (pg 183)*
 2 tbsp natural almonds

Daily Total: 1500 calories

Voila Vinaigrette

This basic recipe for a vinaigrette that contains monounsaturated fats will become a staple for adding personality to your salads. Experiment with the basic formula and you can create a world of possibilities! Keep extra dressing on hand in an airtight container in the refrigerator to use on salads or to brush over cooked meats, chicken, and fish to add a punch of flavor.

1 tbsp	vinegar (white wine, red wine, balsamic, cider, rice wine etc.)
1/2 tsp	Dijon mustard
1/4 tsp	salt and freshly ground pepper
1/4 cup	extra virgin olive oil or canola oil

Stir vinegar, mustard, salt, and pepper until well mixed. Whisking constantly, drizzle in olive oil. Recipe doubles and triples easily. Makes about 5 tbsp (enough for at least 2 salads).

Try one or two of these suggested add-ins to personalize the salad dressing:

1/2 tsp	minced fresh garlic
1/2 tsp	minced fresh ginger
1/2 tsp	lemon, lime, or orange zest
1 tsp	chopped fresh leafy herbs (i.e. basil, oregano, mint)
1/2 tsp	chopped fresh woody herbs (i.e. rosemary or thyme)
Pinch	crushed hot pepper flakes or colored peppercorns
1/4 to 1/2 tsp	honey, agave syrup, or pure maple syrup
1/4 tsp	grated horseradish or hot pepper sauce
Pinch	ground cayenne, curry powder, chili powder, turmeric, paprika, or cumin

Or, for a brand new flavor, follow one of these substitution suggestions:

Lemon or lime juice for vinegar
Grainy mustard for Dijon
Miso paste for Dijon
Sodium-reduced soy sauce for half of the vinegar

Nutrients per serving: 97 calories, 11 fat, 0 g carbohydrates, 0 g fiber, 0 g protein, 132 mg sodium.

EASY YOGURT DIPS

Vegetable sticks get new life when paired with a flavorful instant yogurt-based dip. Try these suggested combos or experiment with your own favorite calorie-free herbs and spices.

Into 1 cup of Greek or probiotic yogurt, stir in (to taste):
- Minced garlic, chopped fresh mint, and grated cucumber
- Curry powder, ground cumin, and finely grated lime zest
- Minced garlic, finely grated lemon zest, and chopped fresh chives
- Chili powder, chopped fresh oregano, and finely grated lime zest
- Minced garlic, a smidge of whole grain mustard, tarragon, and cracked black pepper

Greek style yogurt is a thick and creamy low-fat yogurt. You can make a similar version by placing fat-free plain or vanilla probiotic yogurt in a cheesecloth or coffee-filter-lined sieve over a bowl. Cover and place the bowl in the refrigerator. Strain for at least four hours or overnight. Discard the liquid that accumulates in the bowl and store the strained yogurt for up to 3 days.

DAY 3

One important way to control calories and sodium is to omit butter on cooked foods. Vegetables can be dressed up with squeeze of fresh lemon juice or a drizzle of flavorful balsamic vinegar to add low-calorie flavor.

Breakfast
1 portion *Chocolate Banana Protein Shake (pg 163)*

Snack
1 cup shelled unsalted edamame (green soybeans)

Lunch
1 portion *Mix-and-Match Big Salad* (**pg 159**)
1 whole grain roll

Snack
1/4 cup *Easy Yogurt Dip (see tip box)*
1 cup sliced jicama
1 cup carrot sticks

Dinner
6 oz grilled or broiled free-range, boneless, skinless chicken breast
1/2 cup cooked brown rice
1 cup steamed asparagus
1 small tomato, sliced and drizzled with balsamic vinegar

Daily Total: 1500 calories

Chocolate Banana Protein Shake

This shake is fast and easy and will keep you satisfied and energized all morning. Experiment with other flavor combinations by using vanilla or strawberry flavored whey protein. Adding the flax seeds or oil will provide a healthy boost of Omega 3 fatty acids.

1	banana
1 cup	plain soy beverage or skim milk
6	ice cubes
1 scoop	chocolate flavored whey powder
1 tbsp	ground flax seeds (or 1 tsp flax seed oil)

Combine all ingredients in blender and blend until smooth and frothy.

Makes 1 serving (doubles easily).

Nutrients per serving: 365 calories, 9 g fat, 39 g carbohydrates, 5 g fiber, 33 g protein, 175 mg sodium. Excellent source of vitamin D, folate, vitamin B12, and calcium.

DAY 4

The bakery section in many supermarkets has a selection of whole grain products. Including whole grains in your diet on a regular basis provides not only a source of complex carbohydrates but also many essential nutrients such as B-vitamins, folate, iron, and antioxidants. Sprouted grain breads such as Ezekial bread are one of my favourite choices because the sprouted grains provide a complete protein source as well as vitamins, minerals, and fibre.

Breakfast
Skinny Breakfast Sandwich * *(see tip box pg 165)*
1 whole orange

Snack
1 kiwi
2 tbsp toasted green pumpkin seeds

Lunch
1 portion *Mix-and-Match Big Salad (pg 159)*
1 whole grain roll

Snack
1/2 cup 1 % cottage cheese
3 wedges cantaloupe

Dinner
5 oz grilled or broiled white fish such as wild Pacific halibut or US farm-raised catfish
1 portion *Spicy Sweet Potato Wedges (pg 165)*
1/2 cup steamed sweet peas

Daily Total: 1500 calories

Spicy Sweet Potato Wedges

These zesty potato wedges are a great alternative to fat-laden French fries. Sweet potatoes are rich in antioxidants and leaving the peel on provides a boost of fiber.

1 tsp	chili powder
Dash	cayenne pepper
1/2 tsp	sea salt (optional)
2	small sweet potatoes, cut into wedges
1 tbsp	canola oil
1/2	jalapeno pepper, seeded and finely chopped (optional)
1	green onion, chopped
1/4 tsp	lime zest
1 tbsp	lime juice

Preheat an outdoor or indoor grill to medium. Combine flour with chili powder, cayenne, and salt (if using). Toss with sweet potatoes.

Lay sweet potato wedges, two deep, in a row on a large piece of nonstick, heavy-duty foil. Drizzle evenly with oil. Fold over foil and tightly seal to make a secure packet.

Place packet on grate and close the lid. Cook, turning often, for 30 minutes or until potatoes are tender and well browned. Carefully open the packet; sprinkle with jalapeno (if using), green onions, lime zest, and juice. Makes 2 servings.

Tip: To prepare the potatoes in the oven, bake the packet at 375°F for 40 minutes.

Nutrients per serving: 155 calories, 7 g fat, 22 g carbohydrates, 4 g fiber, 2 g protein, 601 mg sodium. Excellent source of vitamin A.

EGG WHITE 101

Egg whites are a lean protein source. With only 15 calories per serving and zero grams of fat, 1 large egg white provides 4 grams of protein. Scramble egg whites in a nonstick pan as you would regular eggs. For a nutritious and filling alternative to fast food breakfasts, try this **'Skinny' Breakfast Sandwich:** Top a toasted whole wheat English muffins with 2 scrambled egg whites, 2 slices avocado, 1 slice tomato and 1 slice of part-skim mozzarella cheese.
(1 serving = 325 calories)

DAY 5

By day five you should be feeling a few changes in your body. Keep up the good work with this roster of fresh and fabulous foods. Kashi GoLean is a high fiber, high protein breakfast cereal made from whole grains. Wholesome cereals like this one taste delicious when layered with yogurt and berries to make a breakfast parfait. For a tasty afternoon snack, roll the turkey, lettuce leaves, and cheese into two wheat-free roll-ups.

Breakfast
1 1/2 cups Kashi GoLean cereal
1 1/2 cups skim milk
1 cup fresh strawberries

Snack
2 tbsp *Hollywood Hummus (pg 173)*
1 large red pepper, sliced

Lunch
1 portion *Mix-and-Match Big Salad (pg 159)*
1 whole grain roll

Snack
2 slices oven roasted turkey breast
2 lettuce leaves
1 slice part skim havarti cheese

Dinner
1 portion *Good Times Gazpacho (pg 167)*
1/4 Avocado
2/3 cup (3 oz) cooked shrimp
4 Wasa crackers

Daily Total: 1500 calories

Good Times Gazpacho

This easy to make cold soup can be doubled easily. At only 100 calories per serving, this soup provides a nutritious and satisfying way to conquer hunger pangs any time of the day.

2	vine-ripened tomatoes, coarsely chopped
1/4	yellow pepper, chopped
1/4	seedless cucumber, chopped
1	green onion, chopped
1	small garlic clove, minced
1 tbsp	each extra virgin olive oil and red wine vinegar
2 tbsp	chopped fresh basil or coriander (optional)
	Hot pepper sauce, salt and pepper to taste

Combine the tomatoes, yellow pepper, cucumber, green onion, garlic, olive oil, and vinegar in a food processor or blender. Pulse until finely chopped but not puréed. Blend in herbs (if using). Add hot pepper sauce, salt, and pepper to taste. If time permits, chill for 30 minutes to infuse flavors. Makes 2 servings.

Tip: Use a food processor to make a chunkier soup and a blender to make a smoother soup.

Nutrients per serving: 100 calories, 7 g fat, 9 g carbohydrates, 2 g fiber, 2 g protein, 300 mg. Excellent source of vitamin C.

DAY 6

Extra-firm tofu is a meat alternative that's low in saturated fat and very quick to prepare on even the most time-crunched night. Simply brush slices of tofu with a little *Voila Vinaigrette (pg 161)* and then grill or brown in a cast iron skillet for 2–3 minutes per side.

Breakfast
1 portion *Mediterranean Egg White Omelet (pg 169)*
1 slice whole grain toast
1 grapefruit
1 tbsp honey

Snack
1 apple
1 stick, part-skim string cheese

Lunch
1 portion *Mix-and-Match Big Salad (pg 159)*
1 whole grain roll

Snack
1 Wasa cracker
1 tbsp almond butter
1/2 cup strawberries

Dinner
3 oz grilled tofu slices
1 tbsp *Voila Vinaigrette (pg 161)*
2/3 cup brown rice
2 cups steamed baby bok choy

Daily Total: 1500 calories

Mediterranean Egg White Omelet

This tasty breakfast omelet relies on leftover grilled vegetables for preparation speed and morning convenience. Toss thinly sliced vegetables with a little olive oil or **Voila Vinaigrette (pg 161)** and your favorite fresh herbs. Grill, turning as needed, until tender. Store in an airtight container in the refrigerator for up to three days.

1 cup	pasteurized liquid or separated egg whites
	Salt and pepper
2 tsp	olive oil
1 cup	chopped, grilled mixed vegetables such as zucchini, mushrooms, eggplant, and peppers
1/4 cup	halved cherry or grape tomatoes
1/4 cup	lightly packed fresh basil leaves, chopped
1 tbsp	**Voila Vinaigrette (pg 161)**

Season the egg whites with salt and pepper to taste. Set a medium skillet over medium heat. Brush with olive oil. Add the egg whites, tilting the pan to coat evenly. Cook for 2 to 3 minutes or until eggs are set on the bottom but the top is still moist. Toss the grilled vegetables, tomatoes, and basil with the vinaigrette. Sprinkle one half of the omelet evenly with the vegetable mixture. Use a thin spatula to fold the ungarnished omelet portion over the filling. Cover; remove from the heat and let stand for 2 minutes. Makes 2 servings.

Nutrients per serving: 167 calories, 10 g fat, 5 g carbohydrates, 2 g fiber, 14 g protein, salt. Excellent source of vitamin C and folate.

Variation: Substitute 1 cup baby spinach or arugula for the grilled vegetables.

DAY 7

You've made it through the week! Tonight's entrée is elegant enough to have with company so feel free to double the recipe and invite a couple of friends to dine with you. Otherwise, make sure you celebrate your first week's success on your own.

Breakfast

1 portion *Apple Cinnamon Amaranth (pg 177)*
1/4 cup Greek-style or probiotic yogurt

Snack

2 tbsp *Hollywood Hummus (pg 173)*
1 large red pepper

Lunch

1 portion *Mix-and-Match 'Big' Salad (pg 159*
1 whole grain roll

Snack

2 cups plain air popped popcorn
1 tbsp grated Parmesan cheese
1 tbsp toasted green pumpkin seeds

Dinner

1 portion *Herbed Salmon Packets (pg 171)*
1 cup *Mashed Cauliflower (see tip box page 171)*
1/2 cup steamed baby peas

Daily Total: 1500 calories

Herbed Salmon Packets

Preparing foods in a parchment packet creates a dramatic table presentation. This cooking method also keeps food moist and flavorful without adding a lot of extra fat. Use this method when preparing other types of white fish, shrimp or even boneless, skinless chicken breasts.

2 cups	mixed red, orange, and yellow pepper, thinly sliced
1/2 cup	thinly sliced red onion
2	(5 oz) boneless, skinless, wild salmon fillets
1 tbsp	each fresh lemon juice and extra virgin olive oil
1/4 tsp	each sea salt and pepper
1/4 cup	mixed chopped fresh leafy herbs such as parsley, chives, oregano, basil, dill, or coriander
	Lemon wedges

Preheat the oven to 375°F. Fold two, 14-inch square sheets of parchment paper in half; cut so that each piece is heart-shaped when unfolded. Divide sliced peppers and red onion equally to cover one half of each paper "heart". Place a piece of fish on top of vegetables. Drizzle evenly with lemon and olive oil. Sprinkle with salt, pepper, and an equal portion of fresh herbs.

Fold over the other side of each "heart"; roll and pinch edges to seal packets closed. Place on a baking sheet; bake for 25 minutes. Transfer packets to dinner plates. Being careful to avoid steam, cut packets open at the table. Makes 2 servings.

Tip: Substitute 2 cups of chopped Swiss chard or kale leaves for the peppers.

Nutrients per serving: 300 calories, 16 g fat, 9 g carbohydrates, 2 g fiber, 29 g protein, 351 mg sodium. Excellent source of vitamin C, folate, vitamin B6, vitamin B12, niacin, riboflavin and thiamin. Provides 2.5 g omega 3 fatty acids.

MIXED UP MASH

Traditionally prepared mashed potatoes, although wholesome, can provide a lot of calories per serving. Instead, try mashing up steamed cauliflower. Mash as you would traditional cooked potatoes and add a splash of sodium-reduced chicken or veggie broth for a smooth texture. Dare to compare? 1 cup of this delicious mash contains 40 calories compared to a whopping 233 calories in 1 cup of mashed potatoes prepared with 2% milk and margarine.

DAY 8

You've made it past the half way point! Starting this week with an upbeat attitude will go a long way toward reaching your health goals. Today is a good day to stock up! Make some extra hard boiled eggs, a fresh batch of *Hollywood Hummus (pg 173)* and some extra cooked chicken breast so that meal preparation during the next seven days will be easier.

Breakfast

2 hard-boiled omega-3 eggs
1 slice whole grain toast
1 banana

Snack

1 apple
1 stick, part-skim string cheese

Lunch

1 portion *Mix-and-Match Big Salad (pg 159)*
1 whole grain roll

Snack

2 tbsp *Hollywood Hummus (pg 173)*
1 cup carrot sticks

Dinner

4 oz broiled, baked or grilled free-range boneless, skinless chicken breast
1 portion *Spicy Sweet Potato Wedges (pg 165)*
1 cup steamed asparagus
1 cup halved cherry tomatoes

Daily Total: 1500 calories

Hollywood Hummus

This is a nutritious, multipurpose dip that provides a complete protein source when combined with whole-grain pitas. Love garlicky Caesar salad but don't want all the fat? Blend a portion of this hummus with enough water to make a pour-able dressing and toss with leafy romaine lettuce. If you have a favorite prepared hummus you can substitute it in the menu for this homemade version. Just be sure to look for a hummus that contains no preservatives or additives.

1 can	(19 oz) chickpeas, drained and rinsed
1/2 cup	tahini (ground sesame seed paste)
3	garlic cloves
2 tbsp	lemon juice
1 tbsp	extra virgin olive oil
1/4 tsp	ground cumin
	Sea salt and fresh ground pepper to taste

Combine all ingredients in a food processor. Blend until smooth. Taste and season with salt and pepper if needed. Store in an airtight container in the refrigerator for up to 7 days. Makes 2 cups.

Nutrients per serving (4 tbsp): 192 calories, 11 g fat, 19 g carbohydrates, 4 g fiber, 6 g protein, 291 mg sodium. Excellent source of folate.

Variations:
For roasted red pepper hummus, add 2 roasted red peppers to the food processor before blending.
For herbed hummus, add a handful each of cleaned fresh mint and/or parsley leaves to the food processor before blending.

Pita Chips: For homemade pita chips, cut whole grain pitas into triangular wedges (if using the pocket style pitas, separate into two layers). Spread in a single layer on a baking sheet. Toast in a preheated 350°F oven, turning once, for 10 minutes or until golden and crispy. Store in an airtight container for up to 5 days.

Nutrients per serving (1 pita): 75 calories, 1 g fat, 16 g carbohydrates, 2 g fiber, 3 g protein, 151 mg sodium.

DAY 9

You'll notice that berries turn up often on my 14-day eating plan. That's because berries are rich in nutrients such as antioxidants and fiber that can fight against the signs of aging and prevent disease. When local berries are unavailable during the winter months, rely on individually quick frozen (IQF) fruit that is frozen at the peak of ripeness without the addition of any sugar.

Breakfast
1 1/2 cups Kashi GoLean cereal
1 1/2 cups skim milk
1 1/2 cups fresh strawberries, sliced

Snack
3/4 cup shelled unsalted edamame (green soybeans)

Lunch
1 portion *Mix-and-Match 'Big' Salad (pg 159)*
1 whole grain roll

Snack
1 stalk celery
1 1/2 tbsp almond or peanut butter

Dinner
1 portion *Solid Gold Soup (pg 175)*
1 slice whole grain toast
2 slices reduced fat Swiss cheese

Daily Total: 1500 calories

Solid Gold Soup

This comforting, wholesome golden colored soup can be made in big batches and divided into portions before being frozen to have on hand anytime you need it. Smooth and velvety, it can be packed into your travel mug to sip on the go, yet it is also elegant enough to serve to unexpected guests. Combine this soup with sliced cheese and a piece of whole grain toast and you have a hearty meal that provides 24 g of protein.

1 tbsp	olive oil
1 cup	diced sweet potato
2 cups	diced peeled raw pumpkin, butternut squash, or carrot
1/2 cup	each chopped fresh onion and celery
2 tsp	each minced fresh ginger and garlic
1 cup	sodium-reduced chicken or vegetable broth
1 1/2 cups	water
1 tsp	cider vinegar or lemon juice
	Salt and pepper
2 tbsp	plain Greek or probiotic yogurt (optional)
	Fresh ground nutmeg (optional)

Heat the olive oil in a large saucepan set over medium-high heat. Add the pumpkin, sweet potato, onion, celery, ginger, and garlic; cook, stirring often, for about 5 minutes or until vegetables are tender.

Stir in the broth and water. Bring to a boil. Cover, reduce heat to medium and simmer for 20 minutes. Cool soup slightly; working in batches, purée in a blender or food processor until smooth. Return soup to a clean pot and heat over medium heat until warm throughout. Stir in the cider vinegar. Season soup with salt and pepper to taste. Top each bowl of soup with a dollop of yogurt and sprinkle with ground nutmeg (if using). Makes 2 servings.

Nutrients per serving: 198 calories, 8 g fat, 29 g carbohydrates, 4 g fiber, 6 g protein, 396 mg sodium. Excellent source of vitamin A.

DAY 10

White fish such as halibut or catfish are lean and rich in protein and are easily prepared quickly by broiling, grilling, or browning in a heavy skillet that has been sprayed with cooking spray. Fish is ready if it flakes easily when tested with a fork. Catfish is a firmer textured fish, making it the perfect choice for grilling or stir-frying. For a flavorful side dish at dinner, toss baby potatoes and parsnips with *Voila Vinaigrette (pg 161)* and oven roast until tender.

Breakfast
> 1 portion of *Apple Cinnamon Amaranth (pg 177)*
> 1/4 cup plain Greek or probiotic yogurt

Snack
> 1/4 cup *Easy Yogurt Dip (see tip box pg 162)*
> 1 cup sliced jicama
> 1 cup carrot sticks

Lunch
> 1 portion *Mix-and-Match 'Big' Salad (pg 159)*
> 1 whole grain roll

Snack
> 1 kiwi
> 2 tbsp toasted green pumpkin seeds

Dinner
> 4 oz baked wild Pacific halibut or US Farm Raised catfish
> 1/2 cup roasted baby potatoes
> 1/2 cup roasted parsnips
> 2 tsp *Voila Vinaigrette (pg 161)*

Daily Total: 1500 calories

Apple Cinnamon Amaranth

Amaranth seeds are gluten free and a delicious alternative to oatmeal. Amaranth is a complete vegetable protein and provides essential nutrients such as magnesium, iron, and zinc. With loads of fiber, this complex carbohydrate is worth the calories. For variety, any fresh fruit such as peaches, blueberries or fresh figs can be added to the cereal.

1 3/4 cups	water
3/4 cup	amaranth seeds
1/4 tsp	ground cinnamon (approx.)
1	large apple, cored and diced
1 tsp	honey (or to taste)
	Plain Greek or probiotic yogurt (optional)

Bring the water to a boil in a medium saucepan with a tight fitting lid. Add the amaranth in a slow, steady stream. Stir well and return to the boil. Reduce the heat to low. Cover and cook for 20 minutes or until tender and thickened. Stir in the cinnamon, apple, and honey to taste.

Spoon into 2 servings bowls. Garnish with yogurt (if using) and sprinkle with additional cinnamon. Serve immediately. Makes 2 servings.

Nutrients per serving: 355 calories, 5 g fat, 69 g carbohydrates, 14 g fiber, 11 g protein, 22 mg sodium. Excellent source of magnesium, iron, and zinc.

DAY 11

Today's menu harnesses the nutritional power of green foods. Avocados are filling and contain heart healthy monounsaturated fats. Flip to my *Mix-and-Match 'Big' Salad (pg 159)* for some great suggestions of greens to have for dinner. Wash cooking greens, such as kale, Swiss chard, or collard greens and place in a pot over medium heat. In minutes, they'll wilt using the water that is still clinging to the leaves. Season steamed greens with a splash of lemon juice; it will help your body to absorb the iron contained in the greens.

Breakfast
Skinny Breakfast Sandwich *(see tip box pg 165)*
1 whole orange

Snack
1 apple
2 tbsp toasted sunflower seeds

Lunch
1 portion *Mix-and-Match 'Big' Salad (pg 159)*
1 whole grain roll

Snack
2 tbsp *Hollywood Hummus (pg 173)*
1 large red pepper, sliced

Dinner
1 portion *Balsamic Salmon Ribbons (pg 179)*
1 cup steamed greens such as Swiss chard, collard greens or kale
1 cup steamed broccoli
1/2 cup cooked brown rice

Daily Total: 1500 calories

Balsamic Salmon Ribbons

These delicious salmon ribbons can be made ahead and kept for up to 2 days to serve with steamed greens on the side or over a tossed leafy green salad.

1 tbsp	balsamic vinegar
1 tbsp	olive oil
1 tsp	Dijon mustard
1/4 tsp	sea salt and coarsely cracked black pepper
1/2 lb	boneless, skinless wild salmon fillet
2 tbsp	chopped fresh basil
	Lemon wedges (optional)

Soak 8 wooden skewers in cold water for 30 minutes. Preheat an outdoor grill to medium-high or an indoor grill to high. Stir the balsamic vinegar, olive oil, Dijon, and black pepper until combined.

Thinly slice salmon into 8 long strips; thread onto skewers. Brush evenly with sauce mixture and place on greased grate. Cook for 1–2 minutes per side or until just cooked. Sprinkle evenly with basil. Serve with lemon wedges (if using). Makes 2 servings.

Tip: These ribbons can also be cooked under the broiler for 2 minutes per side.

Variation: Use 1/2 lb boneless, skinless chicken breast or round steak cut into strips. Adjust cooking time as needed until chicken is cooked thoroughly and steak is also cooked thoroughly to your preference.

Nutrients per serving (4 skewers): 234 calories, 12 g fat, 2 g carbohydrates, 0 g fiber, 23 g protein, 432 mg sodium. Excellent source of vitamin D and niacin. Provides 1.3 g omega 3 fatty acids.

DAY 12

By now, you've probably realized that it takes a bit of effort to eat a nutritious and balanced diet everyday; but hopefully you will also have learned some useful shortcuts that make eating well easier, too. When preparing fresh vegetables and fruit as well as protein, it's easy to prepare extra to pack away for snacks and salads. Another tip is to pre-measure snacks such as nuts, cottage cheese, and berries into portion-controlled containers as soon as you unpack your grocery bags.

Breakfast
1 portion *Chocolate Banana Protein Shake (pg 163)*

Snack
1/4 cup *Easy Yogurt Dip (see tip box pg 162)*
1 cup sliced jicama
1 cup carrot sticks

Lunch
1 portion *Mix-and-Match 'Big' Salad (pg 159)*
1 whole grain roll

Snack
2 cups air popped popcorn
1 tbsp grated Parmesan cheese
1 tbsp toasted pumpkin seeds

Dinner
1 cup instant sodium-reduced miso soup
1 portion *Asian Chicken Lettuce Wraps (pg 181)*
1/2 avocado
6 slices tomato

Daily Total: 1500 calories

Asian Chicken Lettuce Wraps

This zesty chicken mixture is tasty on its own but even more satisfying when rolled up into crunchy lettuce leaves for a Korean-style wrap.

1/2 lb	boneless, skinless free-range chicken breast
1 tbsp	white miso paste and water
1 tbsp	each minced fresh ginger and fresh lime juice
1	garlic clove, minced
Pinch	hot pepper flakes
1 tbsp	canola oil
1 tsp	each toasted sesame oil and toasted sesame seeds
12	large leafy lettuce leaves
1 cup	each shredded carrot and diakon (white radish)
1/2 cup	each chopped green onion and lightly packed coriander leaves
	Lime wedges

Place the chicken in the freezer for 30 minutes so that it is easier to slice thinly. Stir the miso paste with the ginger, lime juice, garlic, and hot pepper flakes. Slice the chicken breast into very thin strips. Toss with the miso mixture.

Heat the canola oil in a large, heavy skillet set over medium-high heat. Add the chicken pieces. Stir-fry for 5 to 7 minutes or until chicken is browned and cooked though. Remove from the heat; toss with sesame oil and seeds until coated.

Serve the chicken, piled on a platter with lettuce leaves, vegetables and herbs on the side to make individual lettuce wraps. Serve lime wedges on the side to squeeze over wraps. Makes 2 servings.

Nutrients per serving: 196 calories, 12 g fat, 16 g carbohydrates, 5 g fiber, 9 g protein, 400 mg sodium. Excellent source of folate, vitamin A, and vitamin C.

DAY 13

Keep going strong, right until the end! Today's menu is satisfying and delicious and features a vegetarian option. Health experts recommend eating meatless meals as part of a balanced weekly diet to reduce your intake of saturated fat. Studies show that those who eat vegetarian foods often also consume more fiber and antioxidants than their meat-eating counterparts.

Breakfast

1 portion *Mediterranean Egg White Omelet (pg 169)*
1 slice whole grain toast
1 whole grapefruit
1 tbsp honey (optional)

Snack

3 tbsp toasted sunflower seeds
1/2 cup carrot sticks

Lunch

1 portion *Mix-and-Match 'Big' Salad (pg 159)*
1 whole grain roll

Snack

2 slices oven roasted turkey breast
2 leaves lettuce
1 slice part-skim Havarti cheese

Dinner

1 portion *Quinoa & Veggie Bowl (pg 183)*
1 piece Light Baby Bell cheese

Daily Total: 1500 calories

Quinoa & Vegetable Bowl

Quinoa is a tiny bead-shaped grain. Native to South America, this complex carbohydrate is high in protein and fiber. Called an ancient grain, quinoa is actually the seed of a leafy plant related to spinach. Quinoa provides magnesium and iron as well as beneficial phytochemicals (plant compounds that are linked with disease prevention and good health). For a fancy presentation, scoop the pilaf into radicchio or Belgian endive leaves.

1/2 cup	quinoa
2 tbsp	olive oil
1	onion, finely chopped
1	garlic clove, minced
1 cup	each diced butternut squash and red pepper
1 tsp	chopped fresh thyme leaves
1 tbsp	each balsamic vinegar and fresh orange juice
1 tsp	grated orange peel
1 cup	sodium-reduced chicken broth or water
2 cups	chopped rapini (broccoli rabe), Swiss chard or kale

Toast the quinoa in a heavy skillet set over medium heat for 2 to 3 minutes or until lightly browned. Transfer to a bowl. Reserve. Add the oil to the skillet. Add the onion, garlic, squash, red pepper, and thyme. Cook, stirring often, for 5 minutes.

Add the quinoa, vinegar, orange juice, and peel; stir for 1 minute. Add broth and bring to a boil. Reduce heat and cover. Simmer on low for 15 minutes. Stir in the rapini and simmer, covered, for 5 minutes or until liquids are absorbed and vegetables are tender. Taste and adjust seasoning if necessary. Serve hot or at room temperature. Makes 2 servings.

Tip: Sprinkle with toasted, sliced almonds or crumbled goat's milk cheese for a burst of calcium.

Nutrients per serving: 344 calories, 11 g fat, 55 g carbohydrates, 8 g fiber, 12 g protein, 370 mg sodium. Excellent source of vitamin A, vitamin C, folate, magnesium, iron, and zinc.

DAY 14

Congratulations! You're on your way to a more vibrant, confident, and healthy lifestyle. After this two-week regime, you can pick and choose from these meal suggestions to create a menu that works for you. Apply what you've learned during the last two weeks to help you to choose healthy ingredients and recipes to use in your home cooking.

Breakfast
1 cup prepared oatmeal
1 cup mixed berries
1 1/4 cups plain Greek or probiotic yogurt

Snack
1 Wasa cracker
2 pieces smoked salmon or lox
2 tbsp fat free cream cheese

Lunch
1 portion *Mix-and-Match 'Big' Salad (pg 159)*
1 whole grain roll

Snack
1 cup fresh pineapple chunks
2 tbsp walnut halves

Dinner
1 portion *Shrimp and Edamame Stir-Fry (pg 185)*
1/2 cup cooked brown rice

Daily Total: 1500 calories

Shrimp and Edamame Stir-fry

When combined, shrimp and edamame create a colorful, protein-rich stir fry. Frozen, shelled edamame is available in many supermarket freezer aisles and is one of my favorite convenience legume products. Lower in salt than canned legumes, these pre-cooked beans can be tossed into stir-fries, salad, soup, and stews to add a source of fiber and protein.

1/2 lb	peeled, de-veined shrimp
1 tbsp	olive oil
1 cup	frozen, shelled edamame (green soybeans), thawed
1/2 cup	each chopped red and yellow peppers
1 tsp	dried thyme leaves
2	garlic cloves, minced
1	lime
1/2 tsp	each sea salt and cracked black pepper

Heat the oil in a heavy skillet set over medium-high heat. Add the shrimp, edamame, red and yellow peppers, thyme, and garlic.

Stir-fry for 5 minutes or until shrimp is bright pink. Meanwhile, halve the lime and juice one half. Stir lime juice, salt, and pepper into shrimp. Taste and add more lime, salt, or pepper as necessary. Slice remaining lime into wedges. Garnish with lime wedges on the side. Makes 2 servings.

Tip: To thaw shrimp and edamame quickly, rinse each food separately under cold running water until all ice crystals are gone.

Nutrients per serving: 309 calories, 13 g fat, 18 g carbohydrates, 5 g fiber, 32 g protein, 712 mg sodium. Excellent source of vitamin C and iron.

ACKNOWLEDGEMENTS

THIS IS MY FIRST BOOK SO AS YOU CAN imagine, I have many people to thank. To the team at Key Porter, thanks for believing in me and giving me this opportunity. Suzanne, you're an awesome co-writer and a great teammate. To the Birnboims (Jason, Ronnie, and Roy) who helped in making this possible, thank you for your generosity and support. To Paul Alexander, you're a kick ass photographer and an even better friend.

To Bruce, Vanessa, Jodi, Julia, Joel, Marcus, Niki, Mr. Adam, my sister Maurine and, of course, Laurence—you guys are the best sounding boards a person could ask for and a tireless support system. To anyone I haven't mentioned by name that touches my life every day —thank you for everything, you're not forgotten. To Mark and the team at the Yorkville club, you're my home away from home. Last but not least to all my clients, thank you for letting me pick your brains and opening up to me—it is because of you that I sought to share this with everyone.

Whoooo!

ROCK STAR PERSONAL TRAINER WORK SHEETS

Use this to record your RMR, BMI, your body-fat percentage, weight, and measurements at three stages: prior to starting, after the 14-Day Rock Star Boot Camp, and when you reach your target.

ROCK STAR PERSONAL TRAINER WORK SHEETS

		Before Program
RMR[1, 2]	Kilograms =	$0.4535 \times$ number of pounds =
	Centimeters =	$0.3937 \times$ number of inches =
	RMR =	
BMI[3, 4]	Weight (lbs.) ÷ Height (inches) =	
	Result ÷ Height (inches) x 703 =	
% Body Fat[5]		
Weight		
Measurements	Bust	
	Chest	
	Right Arm	
	Left Arm	
	Waist	
	Hips	
	Right Thigh	
	Left Thigh	
	Right Calf	
	Left Calf	

After 14-Day Rock Star Boot Camp	When Target Reached!
0.4535 × number of pounds =	0.4535 × number of pounds =
0.3937 × number of inches =	0.3937 × number of inches =

NOTES:

1. Women: RMR = 655.1 + (9.563 × weight in kilograms) + 1.850 × height in centimeters) - (4.676 × age).

2. Men: RMR = 66 + (13.7 × weight in kilograms) + (5 × height in centimeters) - (6.8 × age in years).

3. Divide weight in pounds by height in inches. Divide by your height in inches a second time then multiply by 703.

4. Results: less than 20 (could be underweight), 20-25 (normal), 25-27 (overweight unless you have an athletic build), 27 (very overweight). Please consult physician before starting Rock Star Boot Camp if under 20 or over 25.

5. Measure your bust (at the nipple line); your chest (right under your bust); each arm (at the widest circumference of the upper area between your shoulder and elbow); your waist (at its smallest part); your hips (at the widest part when your feet are together); each thigh (at the largest area); and each calf, again (at the largest area widest point).

ROCK STAR MOTIVATIONAL MINUTES

Use this to record your feelings about yourself, your body, and your life. You can record your mojo-boosting mantras and other inspirational thoughts.

12 Questions:	Before Program	After 14-Day Rock Star Boot Camp	When Target Reached!
How do I feel right now?			
How do I think/feel I look?			
What is one thing I like about myself?			
What is one thing I would change?			
How are things going in my life?			
What have I done recently that was great?			

	Before Program	After 14-Day Rock Star Boot Camp	When Target Reached!
What have I done that I could have done better?			
What am I doing to improve?			
Am I pleased with my results so far?			
Do I understand that I am a work in progress?			
What is my mantra & personal motivator?			
Do I know this is part of my road to success?			

ROCK STAR THREE-DAY FOOD DIARY

Keep a careful record of what and when you eat, noting all psychological and environmental triggers and how you felt emotionally and physically if you binged.

Food:	Day 1	Day 2	Day 3
Breakfast			
Snack			
Lunch			
Snack			
Dinner			
How did I feel today?			
Was I on my menstral cycle?			
Did I cheat today?			
What happened (mentally, physically, or environmentally)?			

ROCK STAR GROCERY CART

Here is your personal shopping list created using the Rock Star food principles.

List:	1	2	3	4
Clean Protein				
Complex Carbohydrate				
Fiber				
Fruits				
Vegetables				
Nuts & Seeds				
Herbs				
Water (fluids)				

ROCK STAR ULTIMATE CARDIO AND POWER MOVES MIX MASTER

Once you have completed the 14-Day Rock Star Boot Camp, you can design your own treadmill intervals and resistance circuits.

Date: _____

Cardio Routine: _____

Type: _____

Time: _____

Heart rate: _____

Notes: _____

_____

_____

Exercise Routine:	Power moves (type)	Repetitions	Resistance (lbs)	How I feel?	Other note
Move 1					
Move 2					
Move 3					
Move 4					
Move 5					
Move 6					
Move 7					
Move I created:					
Stretch (check when done)					

ROCK STAR PERSONAL CHOICE PLAYLIST

Make a list of your favorite make-you-move songs, and any new one that you may hear on the radio or at a friend's place. Download, download, download.

Artist	Track	Cardio/Exercise	Makes me feel?

Artist	Track	Cardio/Exercise	Makes me feel?

Artist	Track	Cardio/Exercise	Makes me feel?